NATURAL HEALING

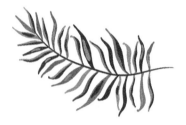

TECHNIQUES

GET WELL & STAY WELL

WITH ASIAN BIO-ENERGETIC THERAPY

JOANNE KLEPAL

with CORY CROYMANS

Live Your Yellow Brick Road LLC

Copyright ©2019 Joanne Klepal

All rights reserved.

Print ISBN: 978-1-73391-340-9

eBook ISBN: 978-1-73391-341-6

www.liveyouryellowbrickroad.com

GRATITUDE

I am grateful for/to:

My friends and family who have supported me along my journey.

The teachers and human angels who help me along my path, and for giving me a good kick every now and again.

My healthy mind, body, and soul.

Mother Nature for providing all we need.

The person I've been, the person I am, and the person I will be.

All of life's experiences, good and bad, as they are all lessons to improve.

Grateful for the moments of just knowing.

Our divine source.

My ABET sisters and brothers.

Madeleine Innocent, for her foreword which is so spot on with the messaging of this book.

The authors of *The New Detox Bath,* Rand Khalil and Lina Baker, for use of the term "Detox Bath".

Although I've not had the privilege of meeting Dr. Thanh Van Le, I'm grateful to him for sharing his experience and knowledge, and for the creation of Asian Bio-Energetic Therapy.

Cory Croymans for expanding upon Dr. Le's Asian Bio-Energetic Therapy and continuing to teach into her seventies. For her continued curiosity to learn and develop all things natural, and for her contributions and experience to the making of this book, including her reviews of my early drafts.

MY JOURNEY AND WHY THIS BOOK

I never dreamed that at fifty years young I'd find myself sitting in Thailand, in a wood house where you can see the floor below you through the planks and hear animals running back and forth in the roof above. In a city I'd never heard of until last year, listening to the birds sing, walking in a garden every day and trying to guess what it is that smells so deliciously sweet, all while writing a book. How did this come to be?

From an early age, I always had something in me that wanted to help others. When I was about eight years old, I remember seeing some younger children hurt themselves in the playground and I immediately ran over to help. When I was about nine, I couldn't stop crying while watching the TV miniseries *Roots* as I felt so bad for the people being mistreated, and just wanted to help those who had been hurt in the past.

Later and throughout my corporate life, I enjoyed mentoring and helping employees develop their skills and watching them grow and blossom in the direction and into the person they desired.

But still, how did I end up here?

Like many, my childhood was far from perfect. I witnessed and experienced physical, emotional, and sexual abuse, lived in foster care, was surrounded by alcoholism, and you might guess, came from a financially poor environment.

Whether a result of my upbringing or not, I knew from an early age that I wanted to "progress", improve my circumstances, be a better person, and have some sense of "financial" security.

I had no idea what that looked like, however there seemed to be an ingrained societal belief that in order to progress, in order to become financially secure, you needed to go to university and gain steady employment, and I thought I was doing well when I found myself diligently on this path.

And then one day, I realized I was unhappy with certain aspects of my life. I thought I had broken the pattern of what I experienced in childhood, until I realized that although I wasn't in a physically abusive relationship, I was in a relationship which had all the same patterns of being in one. I decided I no longer wanted to continue living that way, decided enough was enough, and decided it was time to make a change.

Strangely, at the time, I found myself consciously knowing and aware that this decision was not about the circumstances I found myself in, it was about me needing to change something about me.

This was a major turning point and started me down the path I'm on today. I began turning my focus inward and toward my own personal development. I was introduced to the special gift of

Reiki and I invested in a coach. I began meditating, reading, and attending various seminars and workshops.

The accumulative effects enabled me to have major shifts in beliefs I previously held about myself. Not only did I seem to be consciously unaware of these beliefs, they seemed to be engrained. Beliefs such as:

- I'm not worthy (of love)... to ...I AM worthy...I AM loved...I AM beautiful
- I'm not good enough... to ...I AM perfect as I am
- I'm not deserving... to ...I AM deserving
- I can't do this or be that, because... to ...I CAN do
- I've never been good at... to ...I AM ...I will learn to
- I had a poor education therefore... to ... SO WHAT!
- I don't have a sophisticated vocabulary, I'm not creative, etc., to ... I AM articulate... I have the right words, at the right time, for... I AM creative... I AM an artist... etc., etc., etc.

I found myself writing crazy personal affirmations I would have never previously even dreamed, let alone considered; I had no idea where many of them came from, such as "I am an author," "I am an actor," etc.

I continued my inward focus and step by step, one thing led to another, door after door opened, and then seismic shifts began to occur. One of which, was planning an around-the-world trip which meant leaving a financially comfortable position. It was scary and exciting at the same time. The scary bit came from the old me, and the exciting bit came from the improved me.

I realized this was not about the travel, this was about a shift in my life, a shift in my work, and a shift in me. It was a shift to lead me to the next chapter in my earthly journey. I wanted to learn how to work with energy, learn how to care for my body naturally. I wanted to learn more about how the mind, body, and soul are connected. I wanted to learn tangible skills to help others as I had been helped. It was a shift to better help others along their journey.

I spent two years traveling, mostly throughout Southeast Asia, where I trained, practiced, and taught skills such as Reiki, Neuro-Linguistic Programming, Asian Bio-Energetic Therapy (ABET), Aromatherapy, and other holistic techniques to care for your mind, body, and soul. I even started blogging, which may seem small, but was a big deal for me as it meant moving from being very private to very visible.

While traveling, it had been in the back of my mind to write a book. It was more of a concept then an actual "I want to write a book about such and such." The idea kept lingering, so one night during my Asian Bio-Energetic Therapy training, I went to bed asking, "If I am to write a book, what should it be about?" Lo and behold, I woke up in the morning with the answer, and this book is it. Funny, just a few days ago, I found a mind-movie (an enhanced vision board with sound and movement) that I created just before my travels started, on writing and publishing a book, which until now I completely forgot about.

And so, this, is what led me today, at fifty, writing a book, from someone who once thought of herself as shy and unable to write. By sharing my experiences and sharing some of the wonderful natural and accessible techniques I've learned along the way, my goal is to help empower you to help yourself, so you can live a healthier, happier life.

Now, I can rant and rave about the statistics of diseases our population faces today, even with the billions spent on finding synthetic cures, about how the pharmaceuticals are profit-mongers, about how our politicians and government agencies support the pharmaceutical companies for their own profit. I can rant and rave that the government agencies meant to protect us, don't; instead they support making and keeping us ill. I can also rant and rave about how these same agencies pursue and squash doctors who offer natural therapies and solutions as complements or alternatives to chemicals and prescriptive drugs.

I won't because I expect you already know this, and there is enough information and evidence available elsewhere to support it. What's more important is that you have choices and you are in control of your choices and the changes you wish to see, which means you control the quality of your health.

Having recently traveled back to the U.S., it pains me inside to see so many unhealthy people. It certainly is more visually evident in the U.S. than other places throughout the world. Just step outside your door and you will see people who are extremely obese, people who can barely walk, people who are dependent on scooters and canes to get around, people whose bathroom cabinets are full of prescription drugs, people who are suffering unnecessarily.

This can easily be changed. It can be changed by education and making informed decisions. It can be changed by engaging in, supporting and practicing more holistic and natural techniques. It can be changed by treating the root cause of a health issue, not just attacking a symptom with a drug. It can be changed by treating your whole, interconnected body, mind, and soul. It can be changed by simply making and maintaining good lifestyle habits.

There are so many natural and complementary techniques available to us. My aim is to share and give you a taste of a few techniques that have touched my life along my journey, particularly from Asian Bio-Energetic Therapy.

I expect some of this information will be completely new and you may find you're already familiar with some. Yet you may have found the simplicity of it too simple or too obvious to incorporate into your daily life without understanding the amazing benefits. I found some of the most impactful changes were the easiest to make, and at the same time the hardest, as they were lifestyle choices which I did not want to change out of convenience, such as turning my phone off at night. At the end of the day, this is still an individual choice.

After reading an article written by Ms. Madeleine Innocent titled *Causes*[1], it was clear that Ms. Innocent's message is very much aligned with a key message of this book and with the core principles of many natural techniques and therapies, which is to *find the root cause* of your health problems in order to resolve them! It's worthy of a note here as it truly is another reason for this book.

CAUSES

People often approach me (and I'm sure every other holistic healer, too) for an herbal or similar recommended natural solution for a health problem in their lives or that of a loved one. What they are really asking for is a quick fix.

They have started on the right path of looking for something that won't harm them or their loved one. But it stops there.

What they never ask is "What caused this?" What causes health problems is far more valuable to know and understand than asking for a quick fix. Once you understand what caused the problem, simply addressing that can be the cure in itself. Or a large or important part of it.

Of equal importance, that is never considered in searching for a quick fix, is that you need to consider all aspects of that being's life—the diet, the environment, the treatment to date, and much more. It's not quick. Everything has an influence. Plus, the body is always trying to deal with what's going on.

I do understand that people want to get help. And many want it free of charge. However, this approach is not going to help them much. They're not giving it the consideration that it deserves.

Changing a mindset takes time. Nothing is more important than health. The current medical mindset has invaded the world, but it isn't serving its needs. Look at the escalating chronic diseases. The medical model manages disease. Holistic health care restores health. There is a world of difference.

It's always your choice but make an informed choice. And don't shortchange yourself by looking for quick fixes or questionable advice which may be cheap or free, but without substance. It won't serve you in the long run.

- Madeleine Innocent, Registered Homeopath, Dip Hom, MAHA, MARoH

This book is meant to be informational only and is not meant to diagnose, prescribe, treat, or give medical advice. Most of the techniques are a result of my Asian Bio-Energetic Therapy training and subsequent research and practice. It is not meant to comprehensively cover every single topic or technique from ABET, nor provide ABET training.

Much of this knowledge has been around for many years, in some cases, thousands, so I can't take credit for any originality. My aim is to bring awareness to each technique in an easy and light way, in small bites. You can find extensive scientific research and published materials elsewhere should you wish to take a deeper and more technical look.

As each of our circumstances and needs are unique to us, it's important that you take time to find what works best for you, keeping in mind what is best for us today, may be different tomorrow. If there is anything you are unsure of, use common sense and seek appropriate professional or medical advice according to your needs.

WHAT IS ASIAN BIO-ENERGETIC THERAPY?

"Nature is the physician of disease."

– Hippocrates, 400 BCE

In my early travels around Southeast Asia, when I was making my way to Myanmar (Burma), I wanted maximum flexibility to decide when and where I went and for how long. Most countries have a requirement that you must show proof of your departure before arriving and most airlines ask for this proof at check in, as they have the burden of responsibility to get you out of a country if you cannot provide evidence to immigration upon arrival. I had no clue what my next destination would be, so to meet this requirement, I did a bit of research which led me to Chiang Mai in the north of Thailand.

As Chiang Mai was a short flight from Mandalay, Myanmar, I figured I could regroup there; hey, letting go and seeing where life would take me next, was a part of this journey. Thailand was never one of my original travel destinations, nor had I ever desired to go, and yet it has become the country in which I've now spent the most time, learning so many valuable skills.

While in Chiang Mai, I began searching for places which offered meditation, yoga, and energy work. This led me to Asian Healing

Arts Center. Remember I said one of my goals of this travel journey was to learn to work with energy? Well, their website had a lot of information that resonated with me, such as Asian Bio-Energetic Therapy, Craniosacral Therapy, Aromatherapy, and Reiki. I didn't really understand most of it and I was keen to learn more, so I inquired and booked three ABET sessions.

Before, during, and after my ABET sessions, I was exposed to terms I'd never heard, words that were foreign and alien to me, such as *Bio-Digital O-ring, moxa, magnet therapy, piezo, dampness, Traditional Chinese Medicine (TCM), deviating douche, job tears, urine therapy* and more.

I was astonished to find how much information is out there, if, you know where and what to look for. I learned that Asian Healing Arts Center offered courses in Reiki and Asian Bio-Energetic Therapy once a year. Yes, I signed myself up for both!

I had to figure out how to explain ABET to friends. I didn't fully understand how to explain exactly what it was myself. In my mind, I defined it as a set of Traditional Chinese Medicine principles and techniques which would help keep your body in balance and treat *disease*. But that didn't quite do it justice. If you're from China and other Asian countries, you'll most likely have an idea of what Traditional Chinese Medicine is. I don't recall hearing the term before, so I didn't expect many people I knew to be familiar with TCM either. Additionally, the course also combined other techniques beyond TCM.

After completing ABET training, I reviewed what I learned, and how Asian Healing Arts Center described ABET, and I find I have a much better appreciation for this definition.

Asian Bio-Energetic Therapy is a scientific treatment developed by Dr. Thanh Van Le during a period of more than 30 years. It is a combination of several Asian holistic healing techniques, which are noninvasive, require no machines for diagnoses, and no drugs for treatment. ABET restores the patient's natural energy fields and healing powers, promotes relaxation and healing, and has a positive effect on the emotional, physical, and spiritual well-being.

I did say I had a better appreciation for it, AFTER I studied ABET, so I would understand if you're asking yourself what does that really mean? So, in order to make more sense of this definition, I will walk you through some of the ABET techniques I learned.

Before I dive in, let me first provide you with a bit of background about Dr. Thanh Van Le and Cory Croymans from Asian Healing Arts Center.

DR. THANH VAN LE

Dr. Thanh Van Le[2] was born in Vietnam in 1936. He received his medical education at the University of Wisconsin (U.S.), with a PhD in Oriental Medicine and trained with many spiritual masters in China, Korea, Tibet, India, Japan, Sri Lanka, United States, Taiwan, and Thailand. The combination of his medical training and the healing techniques learned with these masters are what forms the basis of Asian Bio-Energetic Therapy.

Dr. Le taught ABET mostly in Thailand, Vietnam, and Cambodia.

What I found fascinating to know is that Dr. Le also survived five years in a concentration camp in a Vietnam jungle in the 1970s, where hard labor was required with only one bowl of rice a week!

In the mid-1990s, Cory Croymans studied ABET with Dr. Thanh Van Le for three years in Bangkok, Thailand, and as you will soon see, it changed her life in ways she could never have imagined.

Dr. Le subsequently gave Cory permission to teach ABET and has since continued to practice and teach.

CORY CROYMANS AND HOW ABET SAVED HER LIFE

From a young age, I had thoughts, or a romanticized wish, in the back of my mind that I'd love to be able to live with an indigenous culture such as those of the Kalahari Desert, the Americas, or Australia. I wanted to live as they used to, 100 percent off the land, in order to understand and learn to live in a more natural, holistic way, and learn things that are beyond this earth plane in a shamanic, energetic sense. After all, they survived hundreds and thousands of years naturally off the land.

As I was writing this book, it occurred to me that in some small way, this has come to life for me now, albeit in a different form, such as spending time in the Peruvian Amazon, meeting Cory, being exposed to energy work, organic methods, natural ways of taking care of oneself, and more.

In my opinion, Cory has a wealth of knowledge which can be difficult to find these days. She is also one of those people that you either like or you don't; there isn't much in between. She is seventy-one years young and incredibly strong willed. If you can see beyond this, you'll see she has a gigantic heart and the greatest intention to help others.

If you've been to Asian Healing Arts Center, you'll find her wearing shirts and pants with extra-large pockets. You can always be surprised at what she'll pull out to share with you, whether it's a hydrosol or new essential oil that she's recently distillated, a new healthy treat she's found, or anything else that would naturally benefit you at that time.

You'll find her regularly experimenting with new, organic herbs, fruits, essential oils, and more on her property. She generously supports charitable causes, such as the New Life Foundation[3], and includes volunteer work in her Reiki training program.

Cory has lived in Thailand for over thirty-five years and has lived and traveled throughout Southeast Asia for more than forty-three. Here's a bit about her journey, directly from her.

When you look at me, you may think why I should be talking to you about health because I may not look like the best example of a healthy person. Let me tell you why I can.

In 1993, I went for a medical check-up in my home country Belgium. My doctor told me that I would have only five years to live because:

- *My blood pressure was over 200 (normal in Belgium is less than 150).*

- *My cholesterol was 330+ (normal range in Belgium is 150 to 260).*

- *My triglycerides, a type of fat in the body, were 529! A normal range is lower than 160.*

- *My blood sugar level was in the range between 88 and 100.*

- *My blood count was not good and my neutrophil (white blood cell responsible for the body's protection against infection) was high. Both are alarm bells for cancer.*

- *Additionally, I had liver and gallbladder problems.*

That Belgian doctor gave me some of those "new" medicines which almost everyone is taking now (e.g., Zocor, Lipitor), but back then, they were in early stages of FDA approval.

These drugs made me feel so sick that I asked the advice of my friend and doctor when I came back to Bangkok, and this Bangkok doctor told me the following:

"You do not have to take these drugs, if you can change your lifestyle as follows:

- *Stop working sixteen hours per day, seven days a week. Reduce the working hours to twelve (if you can) and do not work on Sundays.*

- *Go to the sea for a long three-night weekend once per month.*

- *Drink at least 1.5 liters of water per day, every day and one extra glass with every cup of tea or coffee.*

- *Start each day with two glasses of water (not cold).*

- *Walk two times per day for 10 to 15 minutes, in the early morning and late evening.*

- *Limit your food intake to one serving at every meal and take your meals on time; three times per day. Do not skip any meal.*

- *Do not eat any pork, or shell foods such as prawns, crabs, and lobster.*

- *Eat more vegetables and nuts. Keep some nuts in your pocket for when you feel tired or "hungry."*

- *Eat foods according to the season and your age.*

- *Do not take any cold drinks, ever.*

- *No ice cream, cheese, or chocolates for a minimum of six months.*

- *No microwaved foods or drinks.*

- *Take dried garlic powder capsules two times per day (not extracts nor pearls, just dried garlic powder in caps). (Don't worry, you won't smell like you ate a ton of it.).*

- *No alcohol whatsoever.*

- *Have regular acupuncture sessions to activate your Qi circulation (four times per month) and do Tai Chi or Qi Gong every day for 10 to 20 minutes.*

- *Stop smoking.*

I did most of what this Traditional Chinese Doctor suggested, and these small lifestyle changes made a very big difference in the quality of my life. Within the next nine months, everything dropped.

- *My blood pressure went from over 200 to 130 and it continues in the range of 120 to 130.*

- *My cholesterol went from 330 to less than 300 and now it's 235. The good cholesterol or HDL, increased from 35 to 88 and the bad one, LDL, dropped from 165 to 83.*

- *My triglycerides dropped from 529 to 404 and now it's at 322; my metabolism improved tremendously.*

- *My blood sugar levels dropped to 90, now 84.*

- *My liver functions cleared up considerably.*

I also had some visible results:

- *I lost 20 kilos, which is so much easier on my heart.*

- *My mobility increased tremendously even though I had broken my back (30 years ago), which prevented me from doing many ordinary things like just picking something up from the floor or working in the garden without being stiffly painful the next day.*

- *I had no more headaches.*

- *I had no more allergies.*

- *I could sweat again; before, I was unable to, even after playing squash for more than an hour with three different people.*

- *In the morning, I could open my eyes easily without them being stuck together.*

- *I no longer got carsick all the time in Bangkok.*

- *I was no longer allergic to house dust, paint, and car exhaust which made my eyes water and affected my vision.*

- *My eyesight improved a lot. So, now I can put a thread in a needle's hole, and I can read my own handwriting easily.*

- *I had no more energy flops which enticed me to take coffees, teas, cokes, or sweets.*

- *I was no longer easily irritated.*

- *My balance became so much better again, so I can ride a real bicycle on the street.*

- *My fingers used to be all crooked and very painful. Opening a jar of anything was impossible, now, I have only one crooked finger left.*

- *My hip joints did not hurt anymore when I walked up the stairs and I can walk very comfortably for two hours (on flat surface).*

- *I had better blood test results.*

How could such small changes affect my health and quality of life that much? This is what generated my interest in Traditional Chinese Medicine because my doctor in Bangkok was a TCM practitioner and acupuncturist.

So, what's the connection to Dr. Thanh Van Le?

The question I had for Cory was, "So how did you come to know Dr. Le?". This was her story.

In 1994, a good friend of Cory's, named Therese, received a phone call from her sister in Los Angeles advising Therese that Dr. Le would be visiting Bangkok. She suggested that Therese go see him as he might be able to help with her hearing. Therese asked Cory if she wanted to come along, and Cory agreed.

After arriving at Dr. Le's office, he asked them both why they came. Cory explained she was accompanying Therese, and Therese explained her reasons and conversed with Dr. Le in Vietnamese which was both of their native tongues.

Cory saw Dr. Le pulling Therese's finger and putting his fingers around both her ears. Therese then said she felt dizzy so, Dr. Le advised her to lie down; she promptly fell asleep for two hours!

While Therese was resting, Dr. Le asked Cory what he could do for her. Even though she had just come along, she advised she had a problem with her middle finger, specifically when working on the computer, it sometimes got stuck, and she was unable to bend or control it.

Dr. Le took Cory's finger into his hands and gently slid his fingers around and down the finger Cory had an issue with. At the same time, he told Cory to take three breaths. He then advised her to bend her finger which she did and found it was now different.

Cory asked Dr. Le what he did, and he responded, "You saw what I did." Cory said, "Maybe not," and that's when Dr. Le invited Cory to be one of his students—with two conditions. First, for the first three months, Cory had to observe what Dr. Le was doing with his patients, six days a week, after her office work. Secondly, she could not ask any questions.

This is how Cory was introduced to Asian Bio-Energetic Therapy and began the next part of her life in the healing arts.

WHY ABET?

"Everything that appears in the physical realm is always connected with energy flow at the invisible level."

– Nan Lu

For the past several years, I've had a physical exam every couple of years and my results always came back showing I'm in top form, and I've always maintained a healthy weight, by Western standards. The doctors were always surprised when I advised, that I took no prescription drugs and rarely any over-the-counter drugs; apparently this was unusual for my age. My physical activity usually varied around my work schedule and where possible, included yoga, Pilates, walking, and sometimes cycling; nothing too strenuous.

Having top scores with my health results was great, however I still felt internally I wasn't fit. For example, I'd feel incredibly fatigued for no reason. I had very irregular sleep patterns. I'd eat, just to eat, even when I didn't feel hungry, and I had developed an irrational fear of heights over the past few years.

I also had a dry cough, for more than 20 years, which sounds like an intense smoker's cough, and it comes and goes, seemingly at random; I'm not a smoker. It was once so bad for three consecutive months, I felt I couldn't bare the soreness in my throat and chest any longer, that I finally broke down and went to the doctor. What did they do? They prescribed medications, steroids, and an inhaler for asthma! I decided not to take them and suffered a bit longer until the cough eventually cleared on its own.

I strongly believe in the mind-body connection. I believe your physical symptoms are sometimes a sign of an emotional imbalance, possibly caused by a past experience and how you associate that experience in your mind. Your regular thought patterns can also cause physical and mental ailments. Have you noticed the thinking pattern of someone who always seems to have a physical ailment or pain?

I remember as a teenager I was asked the question, "Do you think good things happen to good people?" At first, the answer may seem to be an obvious yes. If you asked me today, I'd say not necessarily. Why? Because, if you have negative thought patterns, this is what you will attract. It's not to say bad things don't happen at all or don't happen to those who mostly think positive thoughts. Of course, they will, but how you think and process any event can have a major impact on what you feel, and your physical and mental health.

It's known that we suppress negative emotions and experiences until we are ready to deal with them. If we don't deal with these, they can result in physical or mental symptoms and disease.

It's also known that from birth until about seven years of age, your mind is just observing and soaking in everything around you. It doesn't yet know how to analyze; therefore, you may be storing emotional events from a young age, which you weren't even aware of, that can be impacting your behavior and physical health without you being consciously aware of it.

A good friend used to refer to a four-legged table. The legs being your mind (mental), your body (physical), your emotions (feelings), and your spirit (soul); if one is out of balance or broken, the table is not fully supported, it's unstable and can easily fall or crash.

So, being in what appeared to be good health by Western standards and yet not feeling whole, I was open to trying new ways to ensure I was as vital as I could be. I want to do everything possible to ensure all four legs of my table are strong, sturdy, healthy, and balanced.

This is why I chose to give ABET a try. Before I provide a more comprehensive answer to why I chose ABET, let me walk you through my first experience with ABET as a patient, prior to my training. Don't worry if some words are not familiar to you such as *moxibustion, meridians, O-ring*, you'll learn about these as we move along.

Prior to my first ABET appointment, I was advised that I'd need to commit to three consecutive sessions, or I wouldn't be seen.

Why a minimum of three sessions? I later learned this enables your body to begin rebalancing itself and allows you to notice the cumulative effects of these energy treatments. Depending on a person's condition, additional sessions may be required; remember, I had no major health issues.

I went to my first ABET session curious to know what the best treatment for me was going to be; e.g., Craniosacral Therapy, Reiki, or this thing called ABET. I was advised, first they would assess me, and then determine the treatment. My first session was nearly three hours and my two subsequent sessions were nearly two hours each; all three with various practitioners.

The practitioner started by asking some background information which enabled them to treat me as a whole person and not just any particular symptom I had. I was asked questions such as, reason for being there, my age, my diet, any symptoms, my health history, climates I lived in, my occupation, my sleep patterns, my toilet business, and more.

The practitioner then conducted an initial diagnostic test, using something called the O-ring (BDORT) test. With one hand you form an "o" using your thumb and index finger, and with the other, you touch specific points on your body. What I understood the O-ring test to be, at that time, was a kind of energetic/kinesthetic/ muscle testing to determine areas of weakness or imbalance in the body.

In my case, there were three rounds of testing. After each round, I was asked to do a Tibetan breathing technique, while the practitioner or myself would gently touch an acupoint which was weak. My weak points were then retested, and I was astonished to see these weak points become strong just after doing the Tibetan breathing.

It then appeared that any area still out of balance after the third round of O-ring testing, were the areas requiring additional focus. For me this was the spleen and dampness; both were interconnected.

After my diagnostic test was completed, the practitioner inspected my tongue and what she saw confirmed the results of the O-ring test. I was shocked to see that I had teeth marks on the sides of my tongue that I had never noticed; an indication of dampness in Traditional Chinese Medicine. When was the last time you looked at your tongue; really looked at it?

Magnets were then placed on my weak spots, and I was given a Reiki treatment to allow the body to adjust gently and more deeply to the energy adjustments of the ABET session.

Furthermore, the following lifestyle changes were recommended:

- Drink more water, in my case, three liters per day. The amount of water I required was tested and validated using the O-ring test.

- Drink quality water. After using the O-ring test, I found I would need to drink nine bottles of the current water I was drinking to nourish my body, whereas with a better quality, I only needed to drink two bottles. WOW!

- Eat more cooked green vegetables. No raw vegetables because my spleen was weak.

- Eat three regular meals per day with breakfast between 7 a.m. and 9 a.m., and my main meal no later than 7 p.m.

- Be in bed by 10 p.m.

- Do the Tibetan breathing twice daily.

- Give myself a moxa treatment for 21 days.

- No MSG! It hadn't occurred to me traveling throughout Asia that MSG was commonly used in cooking.

- Stop using my laptop in my lap and on my legs and knees. Are you guilty of using your laptop in bed or on the sofa without any protection between you and the device? Well this causes energy and health problems in the lower abdomen.

- The biggest change of all was to not drink cold drinks, especially in hot climates! This has such an impact on the spleen as you'll see later.

Did you notice in my ABET sessions:

- The amount of time spent with me; three hours in the first session, and nearly two hours in each subsequent session? When was the last time your doctor spent 15 minutes with you let alone one hour or three?

- There were no expensive machines for testing and diagnosing?

- No symptoms were treated?

- No medications were prescribed?

- Only lifestyle changes were suggested?

- If you are familiar with acupuncture, did you notice that no needles were used?

So now, *Why ABET?*

- Many ABET techniques have been successfully practiced over thousands of years.

- It is a natural and holistic approach.

- It is safe.

- No expensive machines are used.

- The focus is on balancing your whole system and root causes, not symptoms.

- No drugs are used.

- Lifestyle changes are easily achievable and, in YOUR hands; you are the master of your destiny.

- It is an easy way to maintain and optimize your health and treat ailments and disease.

- It rebalances your body.

- It enhances your body's own healing potential.

- It can help minimize side effects of medicines.

- It can be used alongside Western medical treatments.

- It is used in outpatient sessions only.

ABET offers a few of the many, safe, natural, and cost-effective techniques you can use to take control of your own health.

As everyone's circumstances are different, every session is individualized, and results can never be guaranteed. Results will vary from person to person, from session to session, and will be based on lifestyle changes you choose to make.

Let me walk you through some of the techniques mentioned above.

WHAT IS THE O-RING TEST?

Professor Omura's Bi-Digital O-Ring Test is so innovative and unusual, yet so simple and elegant, that frankly it strains credulity when first observed in action[4].

The O-ring test is called Bi-Digital O-Ring Test (BDORT). It is a simple, safe, effective and noninvasive diagnostic test which provides feedback from your brain about your body's condition, based on the strength of your fingers.

It is an electromagnetic resonance test discovered by Dr. Yoshiaki Omura in the late 1970s and patented in 1993[5]. As I noted earlier, I see it as a type of kinesthetic/muscle test. In Dr. Omura's testing, it was found that the O-ring had a greater success in detecting early-stage cancers whereas Western medicine typically detects cancer in the later stages when it's harder to treat.

The O-ring test can be used to test many things, for example, remember in my ABET session, my water volume and quality were tested? It can test organ dysfunction. It can gauge if medication is right for your body, and what quantities are best. It can test if a specific food is good for you, where to place your bed in your home, and so much more.

It's so simple. In fact, numerous stories were shared during ABET training about how patients sometimes said, "It's got to be a trick." We had a good laugh later when a friend in the same ABET training used the O-ring test with her mother, and she advised the first thing her mom did was try to see how it worked, thinking it was a trick.

During my ABET session, I was amazed at how simple and accurate the O-ring test was, even with my lack of knowledge of meridian and acupuncture points.

How does the O-ring work?

1. First, the patient, takes the tip of their thumb and index finger and makes an "o" with the thumb and index finger touching each other, tip to tip. The remaining fingers, middle, ring, and pinkie lay flat and relaxed. If you are familiar with mudras, this position is like the gyan or chin mudra.

2. The practitioner, then firmly holds the patient's hand with one hand and with the other hand, makes a ring around the patient's "o" and then firmly and gently pulls.

3. If the patient's fingers stay closed, the area being tested is strong. If they open, the area is weak, indicating a problem.

4. In ABET, the patient's free hand, touches an acupoint, and the practitioner tests if the area is weak or strong using the O-ring.

It's that simple. No expensive medical equipment needed.

By my third ABET session, I found I would inherently know if a point was going to be weak or not, even before the practitioner started the test. This is a common response with patients; they know before you test.

As a patient, one of the benefits of the O-ring is that you are involved in the process and can see what is happening; unlike many experiences where you leave a doctor's office with a feeling that you had no control and no understanding of what was done or why, let alone all the foreign lingo or medical terminology.

So, the O-ring is one of the techniques ABET practitioners use. Now let's look at a few basic Traditional Chinese Medicine concepts and how they relate to ABET.

A SHORT INTRODUCTION TO TRADITIONAL CHINESE MEDICINE CONCEPTS

The body is to nature as a violin is to an orchestra.

The strings are to a violin as the organs are to the body.

For the orchestra to play in harmony all the instruments must be tuned to each other.

If a single instrument is out of tune, the whole sound is dissonance rather than harmony.

– Between Heaven and Earth,
authors Harriet Beinfield & Efrem Korngold

Given that Asian Bio-Energetic Therapy touches on principles and concepts of Traditional Chinese Medicine, it's useful to understand a little bit about these concepts, to better understand ABET. It's meant only to give you an essence of TCM. The study of Traditional Chinese Medicine takes many years and there are plenty of books and programs available should you want more depth on this subject.

Brief History

The earliest traces of Traditional Chinese Medicine go back as far as 5,000 years with Shen Nung recognized as the father of

Chinese medicine. He's the first known person to document plants and herbs with their medicinal properties and is also believed to have introduced acupuncture. There are beliefs that elements of TCM, including acupuncture, can even be traced back to the Stone Age.

The earliest known medical writing *The Yellow Emperor Classics of Internal Medicine* written in the third century BCE, is attributed to Huangdi (Huang-ti), Yellow Emperor, born approximately 2700 BCE. These texts are also known as *Neijing* and the source of development of Traditional Chinese Medicine. Huangdi defined the concepts of Yin-Yang and the Five Elements theory.

Not only has TCM survived thousands of years and evolved with the times, the early foundations are just as solid, safely practiced, and reliable today as in the past.

Did you know that Western medicine used to follow similar principles as Traditional Chinese Medicine? This began to change in the 16th century with the Cartesian philosophy of separation of mind and matter and body, the self and the universe. Since this time, man has looked at the body, mind, health, and environment in isolation, ignoring the impacts to the whole and interconnected implications. The good news is that we are finally starting to see this come full circle.

Basic Concepts of Traditional Chinese Medicine

There are several foundational principals and concepts in TCM, some of which include:

- Human beings are a micro cosmos; a small universe within the larger universe.

- The body is treated as a whole.

- Solve the root cause and symptoms which will disappear.

- The best cure for sickness is prevention.

- Disease is an imbalance or blockage of energy.

- There is a relationship between human activity and the natural environment; everything is connected.

- The best way to live is in harmony with our immediate environment and the universe.

- Everything contains Yin and Yang and good harmony between these energies supports health.

- The body has a natural ability to heal, self-regulate, rejuvenate, and rebalance.

- The body uses electrical impulses to function.

Many of these concepts were influenced by Tao philosophy.

Meridians, Qi, Acupoints, and Yin and Yang

Although modern and quantum science is now confirming and accepting that everything is made of energy, including our bodies, this knowledge has been known for thousands of years in countries such as China, India, Tibet, and others.

In Traditional Chinese Medicine, our bodies have networks of highways or channels in which energy flows. These energy channels are called meridians. Other cultures refer to meridians by different names, such as *nadis* in India, *sen* in Thailand and *channel*, *vessel*, or *meridian* in China and Japan.

The meridian channels form a network which interconnects all parts of our body, physically, emotionally, and spiritually. While these channels are present in the subtle body and invisible to the naked eye, advanced technologies, such as PET scans, can now measure this energy scientifically via our electromagnetic frequencies.

The energy flowing through these meridian channels, known as our vital life force or universal life force, is referred to as *Qi* (pronounced "chee" also written as Chi). Qi flows through our bodies, and through all life, e.g., trees, water, air, animals, our organs, etc. Qi is known as *prana* in India, *Ki* in Japan, and *bio-force* in the West. Qi is the difference between life and death; without it, we would not exist.

Qi primarily comes from two sources. We inherit Qi from our parents at birth. Have you ever heard the expression that somebody has a strong or weak constitution? This can be viewed as the inherited Qi. Qi is also derived from substances in nature such as the food and water we consume and the air we breathe.

According to the Neijing, the purpose of the meridians is to transport Qi and blood, and to circulate Yin and Yang to nourish the body, mind, and spirit. They also carry and transmit information and respond to stimulation. Simply put, meridians regulate energy functions of the body and keep it in harmony.

A blockage in the meridians causes a blockage in energy, resulting in disease, ailments, and pain. A blockage can be caused by a physical, emotional, or mental trauma, such as a sporting accident; bad lifestyle habits, such as junk food; and the environment, such as pollution.

There are places along the meridian lines where energy and Qi collects and rises to the surface of the body. These places are referred to as acupressure points or acupoints: there are 365 primary acupoints.

As an analogy, I think of the London underground tube/subway system where the different lines, such as the Bakerloo, Victoria, and Jubilee, would be your meridians, and the exit points or gates, where everyone comes to surface, would be your acupoints. Any blockage on just one tube line in London, could disrupt and cause chaos across parts of the system or the entire system. This is the same in your body.

Just like the exit gate of London's tube system can be manipulated to control or direct the flow, these acupoints can be manipulated and stimulated to increase or decrease the flow of energy and Qi in the meridians. You'll find this is what acupuncturists do with needles.

Additionally, to correct or fix a problem on one tube line, you may first need to correct a problem on another because they are interconnected. This is the same with your meridian lines and imbalances in the body, as it's all connected.

This is part of what ABET practitioners do. They work to find any weakness or imbalance along your meridians and acupoints using the O-ring test and then help restore balance by using various techniques such as, a special Tibetan breathing technique, using the Piezo activator device, magnets, and moxibustion.

I will further touch on these techniques later. In the meantime, let me share a little more about the meridians.

There are 12 primary meridian lines which run up and down each side of our body and two single line meridians which run up and down the center.

The primary meridians are liver, gallbladder, lung, large intestine, stomach, spleen, heart, small intestine, kidney, urinary bladder, pericardium, and San Jiao (triple warmer). The single line meridians are the governor vessel known as DU, and the conception vessel known as REN.

Ten meridians are directly associated to an **organ and an emotion**, for example the liver is associated to anger, the spleen is associated to worry and overthinking, the lung to grief and sorrow, and so on. I won't cover the detail and function of every organ here; however, I'll briefly cover a bit on the spleen as it plays such an important role and many problems can be traced back to a weak spleen.

Contrary to Western medicine, the spleen plays a significant role and has many functions in TCM. The spleen extracts nutrients from food and drink, transforms this into blood and Qi, and transports this energy to the lungs where it is mixed with the air you breathe to form your vital life force. If the spleen is weak, you may have problems with bleeding, will bruise easily, have low energy and weakness in the limbs, have digestive issues, increased water retention, feel cold, (e.g., hands and feet), and more.

The spleen is also directly related to our thinking and the emotion of worry. A weak spleen may cause excessive worry and impact how well we organize our thoughts and vice versa; too much worry can impact your spleen. Ultimately a weak spleen weakens your immune system.

The meridians are paired in a Yin and Yang combination. According to TCM, everything contains Yin and Yang; your character, your food, nature, weather, and so on.

Yin and Yang are two opposite and yet complementary energies. They are interdependent, and one cannot exist without the other. They are never separate, and within each Yin there is Yang and vice versa. A simple example is night which is Yin, and day which is Yang; one cannot exist without the other and each together create a whole.

Yin and Yang are in constant movement and fluctuation to maintain the ideal state of harmony and balance. Here are some examples of Yin/Yang characteristics:

- Night/Day
- Wet/Dry
- Female/Male
- Rest/Activity
- Stagnate/Movement

In TCM, energy flows through our 12 meridians and organs in two-hour increments via a 24-hour cycle. These times are when your organs function optimally and hold the most energy.

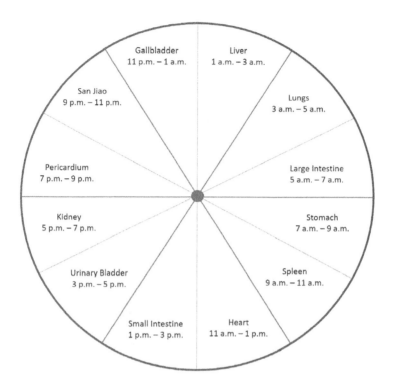

By being aware of these energy cycles, we can align activities in our lives or have a better understanding if something is out of balance. For example, the best time to eat breakfast is between 7 a.m. and 9 a.m. as it's the best time for your stomach to digest. If you regularly wake up between 3 a.m. and 5 a.m. coughing, you may have an imbalance in your lungs, or you may have chronic grief which you need to address. If you regularly feel fatigued at a certain time of day, check to see what organ it's associated with to find the cause. You should ideally be having a healthy stool between 5 a.m. and 7 a.m.; if not, there may be something in your eating habits that you need to address.

Five Elements Theory

The last concept of Traditional Chinese Medicine I'd like to share is the Five Elements theory. The Five Elements theory is used to interpret the relationship between how organs and systems in the body work and communicate together, and the cause and effects of disease of the human body and the natural environment.

Remember I mentioned that one of the TCM concepts is that there is a relationship between human activity and their natural environment and that everything is connected? Remember another concept that our bodies are a smaller universe within a larger one? For me, this is what the Five Elements theory is all about, the elements represent how everything is connected, your body, nature, environment, and so on.

The Five Elements, (fire, earth, wood, metal, and water) are interdependent, and in constant motion and change. For example, there may be a drastic temperature change from one day to the next, from one season to the next, or your choice of foods today wasn't so great, whereas yesterday you may have made healthier choices. Today you may be holding on to lots of anger or stress, whereas tomorrow you may let it go and feel peaceful. If you chose to eat healthy, you'll most likely feel better and have smooth bowel movements. If you're stressed, you're less likely to think clearly and may act irritably.

Here's a visual of some of the characteristics of the Five Elements, our organs, and their associated relationships.

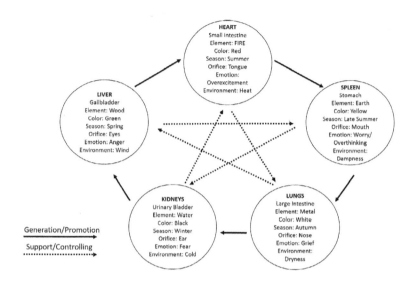

Between the Five Elements, there are two crucial relationships: generation and support. Generation or promotion refers to a growing and nurturing nature. Support or controlling refers to a more restraining force to balance. Without the balancing nature of these relationships, we experience disease.

Okay, enough of the TCM concepts! There is no need to get bogged down on the details of TCM. The information above was to give you a taste of TCM so you can better understand how everything is connected and how it relates to some of the ABET work.

Let me relate some of this to my first ABET experience to demonstrate how it all fits.

How It All Fits

Two big takeaways during my first ABET experience were that I had dampness and a weak spleen.

I had never heard of dampness and didn't really understand it. I eventually found that dampness is a very common term in Traditional Chinese Medicine, whereas I found nothing mentioned in Western medicine.

The descriptions I found indicated that the cause of dampness was a failure to burn off moisture in the body, and the effects could result in feeling tired. Everything consistently indicated dampness was associated to a weak spleen, which was certainly consistent with my ABET diagnosis.

During my ABET session, the practitioner explained that dampness was a form of stagnation or lack of movement in your body's fluids, which make them too sticky, resulting in energy blockages and pain.

So, looking at the connections outlined above, there are four relationships that really stand out for me.

The first, is the relationship between the spleen and damp climate. Wow, what a surprise, all my life I've lived in climates which were either hot and humid or cold and damp.

The second, is the relationship between what the spleen controls, specifically Qi production; energy levels. Earlier I mentioned I wanted to try ABET because, although I'd get top scores on my annual checkups, I'd feel incredibly fatigued, even when I was well rested. Well, a part of having a weak spleen is a Qi deficiency. This makes sense in relation to the fatigue I felt.

The third, is the relationship with the emotions; worry and anxiety. I don't even know where to start with this one as I suspect it could go very far back. Starting from childhood when there was anxiety about siblings and family members being abused, to myself being abused, to worrying if we'd have heat in the winter, and later in adult life worrying about making ends meet, worrying about future security, and so on.

It's probably safe to say that all this worry could certainly have had an impact on my spleen. Of course, it's also a vicious cycle, the more you worry, the more your spleen weakens, the more your spleen weakens, the more worry you have, and so on.

The fourth, is the relationship to the foods I ate. Although I have not described how food fits into any of the above concepts, all foods are Ying, Yang, or neutral. Some of my favorite foods fall under Yin and are ripe for dampness, such as raw vegetables, bananas, watermelon, pumpkin, broccoli, avocado, eggplant, spinach, potato, raw fish/sushi, eggs, and cheese. Oh wait, did I also mention chocolate and ice cream?! I drank hot teas and room temperature water, but I loved to drink iced tea in hot climates and guess what? Cold drinks, period, are a big no-no, for the spleen.

Do you remember some of the recommended lifestyle changes I was given? Here are a couple and how they relate to the above:

- No raw vegetables as they are more difficult to digest which would cause the spleen to work overtime
- No cold drinks as they weaken the spleen
- Daily Tibetan breathing to help improve energy production and circulation, and calms the mind
- Moxibustion to help improve Qi circulation

So, can you see how one thing is connected to another?

Another aspect of what ABET practitioners do, is assimilate information about you, your ailments, lifestyle, environment, etc. With their TCM knowledge, they help you restore your balance and energy, promote self-healing in your body, and help you feel better.

TECHNIQUES TO RESTORE BALANCE AND PROMOTE HEALING

In every culture and in every medical tradition before ours, healing was accomplished by moving energy.

– Albert Szent-Gyorgyi, Nobel Prize Winner

In the previous section, I explained how our bodies have networks of channels (like the lines of the London underground system) called meridians and energy, or Qi, flows along these channels. There are places along the channels where energy/Qi collects and rises to the surface of the body and these are known as acupressure points or acupoints. These acupoints are like the exit gates of the London underground system.

The channels form a network which interconnects all parts of our body, physically, emotionally, and spiritually. The purpose of the meridians is to transport Qi and blood, and to circulate Yin and Yang to nourish the body.

Just like a blockage on the London underground could disrupt and cause chaos across parts of the system or the entire system, the same is true with your body. A blockage in the meridians causes a blockage in energy, resulting in disease, ailments and pain. A blockage can be caused by a physical, mental or emotional trauma, bad lifestyle habits (diet), and the environment (pollution).

Just like the exit gate of London's underground system can be manipulated to control or direct the flow, these acupoints can be manipulated and stimulated to increase or decrease the flow of energy/Qi in the meridians.

ABET practitioners work to find any weakness or imbalance along your meridians and acupoints using the O-ring test and then help restore balance by using various techniques such as, a special Tibetan breathing technique, using the Piezo activator device, magnets, and moxibustion.

Let's start with the special breathing.

TIBETAN BREATHING TECHNIQUE

You can live a few days without food or water, but only seconds without breath. Breathing and how we breathe is important to our health.

Have you ever stopped to pay attention to your breathing or are you only conscious of it when something is drastically wrong, like feeling out of breath or having an asthma attack? Is your breathing shallow or deep? Is it too fast or too slow? Do you breathe with your diaphragm? I remember several years ago when I had my first Reiki treatment, I realized for the first time that I had not been breathing properly; my breath was incredibly short and shallow.

During my first ABET session, after all my main acupoints were tested, I had quite a few weak points; more than 20 in fact. You may recall I had three rounds of testing. After the first round, I was asked to do this special Tibetan breathing technique, while the **practitioner** gently placed her fingers on specific weak acupoints, and transferred energy to me, using the Tibetan breathing technique.

After this was finished, my weak points were retested. I was astonished that some of these points had then become strong, just by doing the Tibetan breathing technique!

During the final round of the Tibetan breathing technique, I, not the practitioner, placed my fingers on specific weak acupoints and it still worked! Each time the breathing technique was used, more of the weak points became strong.

Benefits of the Tibetan breathing technique

- It calms the body and mind.
- It helps to balance the positive and negative energies in your body.
- It helps improve energy production and circulation.
- It increases oxygen in the blood, giving more power to your organs—allowing your body to work better.
- It helps to regulate blood pressure and digestion.
- It can help control your emotions.
- It enables more space for oxygen in the lungs.
- It helps you to breathe through your diaphragm and by doing this, the diaphragm massages your stomach, liver, intestines, thus balancing these organs. This also takes the pressure off the heart, so it doesn't have to work so hard and can focus on the heart's other functions.
- It stimulates digestion and helps remove waste and toxins.
- Increases volume of air per breath by 50 percent.
- Increases red blood cells.

How to do the Tibetan breathing technique

1. Sit or stand up straight or lie down.

2. Close your eyes.

3. Put your left hand, palm upwards, on your left leg. Touch the fingertip of your thumb with the fingertip of your index finger, making an "O," and stretch and relax your remaining fingers. If you are familiar with mudras, this position is like the gyan or chin mudra (see illustration).

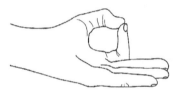

4. Put your right hand, palm inward, just below the belly button, touching this area.

5. Breathe in through the nose, very slowly up the head, down the back until you reach your tailbone.

6. Contract your buttock muscles gently and bring the breath to the front of your body.

7. Slowly push the breath up the front of your body with your belly muscles and then out of your mouth while pursing your lips (like whistling).

Do this technique two times with your right hand just below the belly button and then repeat two times with your right hand on the area where you have pain. This is a total of four Tibetan breathings per session.

It's okay to visualize steps five through seven if you need to, especially with your first attempts.

When can the Tibetan breathing technique be done?

A good place to start is twice per day, morning and evening, and then adjust as necessary; however, you can do this breathing technique anytime you feel like it. I like to do this in the morning before getting out of bed, if I wake up in the middle of the night, and before I go to bed at night.

Try it when you are feeling stressed or tired in the day.

Considerations

- You should not overdo this technique. If you feel you get a dry throat, reduce the frequency.
- If you are not in the habit of breathing deeply, you may feel dizzy the first time(s) you try this technique.
- If you practice regularly, you may find that you release strong emotions or have a sudden desire to cry or burst out laughing. This is okay; you are releasing blocked energies. If emotions come up, acknowledge them and let them go.

One question I had about the Tibetan breathing technique was if there was any significance in the hand positions. The answer is yes. The left hand is the receiving hand, receiving energy. The right hand is the giving hand, giving energy. If you've ever seen Buddha images, have you paid attention to some of the hand positions? If not, take a closer look next time, and you will notice similarities to these positions.

You don't need an ABET practitioner to practice this technique, so feel free to start today. Start slow and easy, and use common sense and judgment based on your own body and knowledge of yourself.

THE PIEZO

During my first and second ABET sessions, I had many weak points, and when tested using the O-ring, my body did not want the Piezo to be used on me, hence the Tibetan breathing technique was used as the first method. By the third ABET session, I had stronger acupoints and my body was now ready for the Piezo.

The Piezo, like the Tibetan breathing technique, activates your meridian lines and the energy which flows through it. It's like giving it a kick start. I was hard-pressed to find information regarding the Piezo, so I will share some of what was presented in the ABET training[6].

The word *piezo* is derived from the Greek word for pressure. In 1880, Jacques and Pierre Curie discovered that pressure applied to a quartz crystal created an electrical charge in the crystal and this is called the piezo effect.

In the 20th century, a Japanese medical doctor, Dr. Takeyoshi Yamaguchi, studied the relationship between electricity and the human body. According to Dr. Yamaguchi, electricity is produced throughout the body from organs such as the heart, the brain, and each individual cell. (Remember one of the TCM concepts was that the body uses electrical impulses to function)?

The body also generates a voltaic current (electric current by chemical action) by muscular contraction and neural stimulation.

This current is used for electro-cardiogram and brain wave tests. This phenomenon is called bio-electricity and plays an important role in maintaining human life. His studies resulted in the invention of the Piezo, which works with a quartz crystal, like how a watch works to generate a low electronic pulse.

Just as acupuncture activates and stimulates points along the meridians with needles to generate electric current to help clear energy blocks, relieve pain, and increase blood flow, the piezo, an electric trigger stimulation, does the same without the use of needles.

To use the Piezo, seek a qualified ABET practitioner, a qualified professional, or have proper training of its use. If the Piezo is used incorrectly, it may cause minor health problems or stop a pacemaker.

MAGNETS

Another tool used by ABET practitioners are magnets. You may recall during my first ABET session, after I was tested three times and Tibetan breathing was used to stimulate my weak acupoints, magnets were then placed on specific weak points. Can you guess why this was done?

Electromagnetic energy is an essential part of our body and we are constantly surrounded by magnetic fields which can have a positive or negative effect on our bodies. Even our organs have pulsing electromagnetic fields. Some of these electromagnetic fields are generated by nature such as the earth and sun, and others are generated by man, such as microwave, x-rays, radio, mobile phones, Wi-Fi, etc. Magnetic fields also have different strengths or frequencies.

As you've been reading here, if our bodies and energy are out of balance due to our lifestyle choices, environmental causes, etc., it can result in pain and disease, and impacts our body's ability to naturally heal itself. Our bodies and magnets produce a negative magnetic field which enables our body to self-heal.

Although magnet therapy has recently gained popularity in Western countries, it has been around for thousands of years; as far back as ancient Egyptian times and is even found in *The Yellow Emperor Classics of Internal Medicine.*

Magnets can be used for many symptoms and diseases, but also small, everyday annoyances. I now use magnets for the small things such as headaches, menstrual cramps, or pain in my hand from using my laptop mousepad. They can even be used cosmetically in place of chemicals such as Botox.

ABET practitioners use negative field magnets to hone in on specific areas and acupoints more deeply.

As with the Piezo, it is recommended that you seek a qualified professional, or have proper training in the use of magnets.

Before I move on to the next tool, I'd like to note that acupuncture, the use of needles, was not a part of ABET training, however some ABET practitioners may be trained and licensed in acupuncture. It's worth a mention because, like the above tools, acupuncture works on your acupoints to activate energy circulation.

MOXA

Moxibustion with something that was called moxa, was incorporated into my second and third ABET sessions. It probably will not come as a surprise that these were more terms I had never heard of.

Notwithstanding that, I thoroughly enjoyed it. Lying down on the treatment table, one practitioner was giving me a Reiki treatment, while another, simultaneously, gave me a moxa treatment; double whammy, I was in heaven. I especially loved the moxa on my lower back, it just felt like I could feel my blood and energy moving.

So, what is moxa and moxibustion?

Moxa is a plant or herb, whose Latin name is *Artemisia argyi* or *Artemisia vulgaris*, also known as *mugwort* and *wormwood*. In Chinese, it's called *Ai Ye* and is believed to have been used by the Chinese even prior to acupuncture. On my way back to the U.S., I made a stop in New York City and was so excited to recognize moxa growing in Central Park!

Moxibustion combines heat with the application of the moxa herb. Moxa is typically used on acupoints and along the meridian lines and can be applied directly or indirectly, at a distance, to the skin.

As previously stated, energy blocks cause disease, ailments, and pain. A blockage can be caused by a physical, mental, or emotional trauma, bad lifestyle habits, and the environment. So, what does moxa do? Surprise, moxa treats and prevents disease by moving energy in the body and along the meridians. Burning moxa close to the skin penetrates the acupoint and meridian.

Benefits[7]

- *Increases production of white blood cells.* White blood cells are important because they protect the body against infection and disease.

- *Increases production of red blood cells and hemoglobin.* Red blood cells are important because they carry oxygen and nutrients around to body.

- *Improves overall blood and lymph circulation.* Blood circulation performs many essential functions such as, carrying oxygen from the lungs to the cells for energy, carrying nutrients to all cells, carrying waste away from the cells, and more. You could not live without blood circulation. Similarly, it's important to keep the lymph system moving to carry nutrition to the cells, take waste away, and to move your white blood cells around.

Moxa is also known to manage inflammation, strengthen immunity, dry dampness, and turn breech babies. Have varicose veins? Have low circulation? Have cold feet? Have an infection? Have arthritis? Have a cold? Have menstrual cramps? Have irritable bowel syndrome? Have an itchy insect bite? Moxa can help with all of these and much more. Every time I use moxa, I feel the energy flowing through my body, as if I can feel the blood running and pulsing through my veins everywhere.

There were two impressive and what I'd call extreme cases of what moxa can do, shared with us in our ABET training. One was of a gentleman who was bitten by a mosquito in India. Over time, the bite turned into a large hole in his leg, nearly one-inch deep, and many doctors could not find what was wrong. After his ABET diagnostics, he was treated with moxa and Cory advised she could visually see the wound start to close on the first moxa session. The wound was completely healed after only four moxa sessions.

The second was of an elderly gentleman located in a remote Thai village where Cory and team volunteered. He lived in a wood house, with three walls and no front wall, and open dirt floors. By Western standards, you wouldn't call this a house; the walls were not even solid. When he was first seen, he had cotton wool wrapped around his feet and was unable to wear shoes or even walk. When the wool was removed, there was a significant amount of puss coming out and three large, open wounds. He had been living like this for a significant amount of time.

He was shown how to apply moxa and advised to do this every day, several times if possible. When the volunteers returned two weeks later, the wounds were completely closed.

These extreme cases demonstrate the wonders of moxa.

It is recommended that you seek a qualified TCM doctor, ABET practitioner, acupuncturist, or other qualified professional, or have proper training in the use of moxa. Overuse of moxa can have negative implications, and is not recommended on certain acupoints if you are pregnant.

The Tibetan breathing technique, the Piezo, magnets, and moxa are just a few of the tools ABET practitioners use to help balance your body and promote its self-healing process by regulating and normalizing the energy flow along your meridian channels.

DETOX BATH

The status of civilisation among any race of people is measured to a very considerable extent by their use of water.

It is a fact that the high quality of culture achieved by Egypt, Athens, Rome, Jerusalem, Cartage, Alexandria, and other great centres of the ancient world went hand in hand with a liberal supply of water.

– Benedict Lust,
"Fountain of Youth or Curing by Water", 1923

It is well known that the use of hydrotherapies and water goes back to ancient cultures and civilizations. After having spent more time researching the next technique, it seems all roads lead to the same resources in more recent history, which is Louis Kuhne and France Guillain.

This technique was recorded first by Louis Kuhne. If you read his story in his book, *The New Science of Healing*, published in 1917, it sounds as if you are reading a story from current day.

Kuhne explains that both his parents had medical conditions which after seeking much medical assistance in the conventional sense, failed to help either of them. His father had cancer. Kuhne subsequently developed cancer himself and after being treated unsuccessfully by conventional doctors, he began looking for natural methods. This eventually led him to develop the friction hip and friction sitz baths.

This was further developed by others and known as the deviating douche, derivative bath, and detox bath[8]. I will mostly refer to this as the detox bath going forward.

After Kuhne succeeded in alleviating his own symptoms, he opened his own clinic in 1883 to help thousands of others. He explains how many patients came to his clinic as a last resort when all other conventional treatments were also unsuccessful for them, and there seemed to be no hope. In his book, Kuhne outlines the results his patients experienced with friction hip and friction sitz baths in so many different illnesses and diseases such as measles, scarlet fever, diphtheria, small pox, whooping cough, gout, sciatica, rheumatism, curvature of the spine, and so much more[9].

I liked that Kuhne took a holistic and whole approach with his patients. For example, he not only applied his hydrotherapy methods, he also counseled patients on their dietary needs.

Kuhne's friction sitz bath was further expanded on by France Guillain. Ms. Guillain, born in Polynesia and educated in France in her adult life, spent 17 years sailing the globe with her five daughters, mostly on her own. She describes that not only were there no radar or satellites on her sailboat, she was visiting countries where the few medical supplies she did carry, could not be replenished.

She suffered from painful finger arthritis in both hands, and after visiting numerous doctors and specialists, the only thing she was given was anti-inflammatory medication which she decided not to take after learning it would not heal her problem. In one of her ports of call, she was told of a friend's girlfriend who had a similar problem and who "did something to cleanse the body." Guillain was told to take a bucket of seawater, twice a day, and cool down her genitals for up to 30 minutes.

Guillain tried this and found after a few days, she felt better, slept better, was more energetic, and the swelling disappeared. She explains years later when she broke a finger, her doctor was surprised to find her previous arthritis completely healed, which was opposite of what would have been expected, to get worse over time. She later realized that her joints became more flexible, as a result of removing fat and toxins[10].

What is the detox bath and how does it work?

Did you know that the groin area is one of the areas of the body with the highest concentration of nerves? Did you know that this area also houses main arteries?

The detox bath is a method to cool down your genitals, to stimulate the body to remove toxins and excessive fats. When your body absorbs toxins, they are sent to the extremities of your body (e.g., feet, hands, head) where they cannot be eliminated, and this overworks your body's systems. The detox bath helps increase the elimination of these toxins.

Of course, toxins can be anything from processed foods, pesticides, chemicals in the air fresheners we breathe or the candles we burn, environmental pollution, chemicals in moisturizers and makeup we put on our skin, chemical cleaning products, electrical devices, and much more.

Guillain explains how the fascia system is associated to fats and toxins and the how the detox bath helps to eliminate them; I'll summarize my understanding very simplistically[11].

The fascia system is a very thin, transparent membrane with billions of channels, which circulate throughout our entire body. The fascia can store fats and toxins. Some fats are good, for example, brown fats act as a reserve in case you stop eating, and to protect us against cold or warmth. Some fats, of course, are not so good; the fascia stores both.

If the fascia does not circulate well, it is unable to eliminate what our bodies don't need. Much like clogged pipes will cause your sink and toilet to back up, the fascia and our bodies will become overburdened and clogged, resulting in negative health implications. So, it's important that the fascia is working well to help eliminate toxins and fats, which can be done by cooling our genitals and applying friction.

Benefits

As the detox bath helps remove toxins and excess fat from your body, it better enhances your body's ability to self-heal and regulate.

Kuhne, Guillain, and R. Khalil and L. Baker the authors of *The New Detox Bath*[12], outline many stories of how people have benefited from this technique, such as:

- Elimination of toxins
- Improved digestion
- Improved bowel movements
- Reduced inflammation
- Removal of excessive fat and cellulite
- Improved sleep quality
- Increased energy
- Increased metabolism
- Loss of body volume and increased body tone
- Improved complexion

How to Perform the Detox Bath

There are three primary methods to performing the detox bath[13].

Bucket Method

The first is to sit over the bathtub or toilet with a bucketful of cold water.

Dip a hand glove, sponge, or cloth into the cold water and gently brush over either side of your genitals downward to the perineum for up to 20 minutes, two times per day.

For men, at a minimum, you can apply the glove, sponge, or cloth to the tip of the penis. Optionally, you can also apply this to the length of the penis and testicles, so long as it is not painful.

Hand-Held Sprayer

What I love about being in Asia is having access to a hand-held sprayer device near every toilet as it allows you to clean yourself after taking a wee or poo. This feels much fresher and more sanitary than using just toilet paper.

This hand-held sprayer device can also be used for a detox bath. Like the bucket method, use the sprayer device to spray over the side of your genitals for up to 10 minutes, two times per day, or just an extra minute or two each time you use the toilet.

If you have a showerhead connected to a long enough hose, you can use this in a similar way in the tub/shower. Of course, if you have an actual bidet, you can use this as well.

Especially for the bucket and hand-held sprayer methods, you may choose to adjust the amount of time based on your needs.

Cold Gel Pack

Place a cold gel pack or small bottle of water in the freezer and when ready, place this on your genital area for one hour. The length of time for the cold pack is longer because you are only applying cold temperature with no friction.

You should remove the pack when it gets warm. I find it handy to have an extra pack in the freezer.

Take sanitary precautions such as putting your gel pack in a sealed bag in the freezer and wrapping the bottle with a towel.

This method is super convenient around the house as you are sitting or lying down, working on your laptop, watching TV or reading.

Considerations

- Keep your body warm.
- Sit down and ensure you are in a comfortable position.
- Use water that is cooler than your body temperature, like cold tap water. It should be comfortable and not hurt, so adjust accordingly.

- Don't allow the cooling water to run down your legs, as it would when taking a shower.

- Use a smooth glove, sponge, or cloth.

- Wait at least an hour and a half after eating a meal to have a detox bath.

- Take sanitary and hygienic care with any option you chose.

- Avoid during menstruation.

I was curious to understand the reasons to avoid during menstruation, so I contacted the authors of *The New Detox Bath*, and they advised to avoid for hygienic reasons, and that cold water on the groin during menstruation could increase the intensity of any related cramps.

Remember that as you release toxins from your body, it is natural for you to initially experience headaches, nausea, tiredness, skin rashes, and diarrhea. Be aware of this and be kind to yourself.

Today, we are marketed many kinds of expensive detox methods, such as pills; I know, I've been there! The detox bath is a free, easy, and natural method to remove toxins from your body.

Staying on the lower part of our body, let's move to our next technique.

DIVINE NECTAR

A crucial fact that we have overlooked in this era of modern medicine is that the body itself has the innate natural ability to adapt and change to new disease influences, but chemical drugs do not.

– *Your Own Perfect Medicine,* author Martha M. Christy

Over the past century or so, particularly in the West, not only did we "throw the baby out with the bath water" when it comes to natural therapies, we've come to believe that Western or modern medicine can cure all, even when it has shown otherwise.

- How easy has it been for you or those you know to pop a pill for every ailment?

- Have you ever stopped to look at your medicine cabinet; does it look like you can open your own pharmacy?

- How many of you are looking for the miracle cure and quick fix for the years of abuse and neglect you put your body through?

Many live their lives as if a pill a day, will keep their pain and disease away.

I remember the first time when I was watching television in the U.S. and I noticed every other commercial was for some drug or for some ailment or another. I cracked up when I heard the multitude of side effects for the drug being promoted; these side effects took the greater portion of the advertisement. I remember thinking, the list of side effects surely wasn't worth it; you're trading one issue for a multitude of others, which sound much worse!

Would you be interested in another natural therapy which is easily accessible and customized to your individual needs? A natural therapy which has a history that can be traced back centuries to societies in ancient Egypt, China, India, and Aztec culture? A solution which has had vast amounts of research, study, and data collected more recently over the past century or so? If so, read on with an open mind and a sense of curiosity.

I was first exposed to the information I'm about to share during my first ABET session. A few months later, I was exposed to the concept again in India while I did an Ayurvedic *Panchakarma* cleanse. The topic was subsequently covered in ABET training and I've continued being educated by further research and use.

It's called, *urotherapy*, also known as urine therapy, urinotherapy, uropathy, auto-urine therapy, or AUT; for simplicity, I will abbreviate this as UT.

What is urotherapy?

Urotherapy is reabsorbing your own urine externally or internally, such as massaging it into your skin or drinking it.

Yes, you heard and read right! If your initial reaction is shock, wouldn't this be due to the fact we're trained to believe our urine is unclean? Did you know the fluid that you and I floated in as a fetus was mainly composed of urine? That, as a fetus, we would breathe it into our lungs?

Did you know that urine is used in making cosmetics and skin creams? Yes, the stuff you apply on your face. It is also used in manufacturing hormones and drugs.

Don't think urine is important? In *Your Own Perfect Medicine*, author Martha M. Christy outlines an article published by *Hippocrates Magazine* in 1988 that describes a company that designed a special filter to collect urine from portable toilets, what we call porta-pottys. It stated the market for ingredients found in urine was $500 million per year. If that was in 1988, imagine what that figure is today!

Benefits

Research has shown that UT has been successful in treating numerous aliments including allergies, asthma, burns, cancer, candida, cystitis, diabetes, eczema, gonorrhea, gout, HIV, inflammation, infections, migraines, polio, rabies, tuberculosis, tumors, viruses and much more. It also shows it works as an antibacterial and antiseptic, improves nervous disorders, boosts the immune system, and works to detoxify.

Christy's story is quite fascinating. She describes her own long-term ailments which started in her youth and included chronic pain and fatigue, endometriosis, tumors, internal bleeding, constipation, hemorrhagic cystitis, pelvic pain, yeast infections, thyroid problems, and more. She had seen multiple doctors, specialists, taken numerous prescription drugs, had multiple operations, and tried natural therapies, all without any significant or lasting success.

In her early forties, she was introduced to UT and states she got immediate relief from her constipation and fluid retention, and within one week her severe abdominal and pelvic pain disappeared. Shortly after that, other issues began to disappear or heal, such as her chronic cystitis, yeast infections, food allergies, and digestive problems, and her energy increased. A few months into the UT, she rarely experienced colds, her hair grew back, and she was able to resume working[14].

To better understand why UT is so beneficial and successful in relieving many health problems, let's look at what urine is and is not.

How does UT work?

Do you think that urine is waste and poisonous? It's not. It's made up of 95 percent water, and the remainder is urea and mixture of nutrients/vitamins, minerals, salts, hormones, and enzymes.

Are you asking yourself how is urine good for us if we pass it? I'll try to simplify a very complex process. When you ingest food, it's broken down in the stomach and intestines into small molecules. These molecules are passed into the bloodstream. The blood circulates the molecules and other essentials such as nutrients, enzymes, and hormones throughout the body.

The blood makes its way to the liver where toxins are removed. The good stuff stays, the bad is excreted. The good, purified blood then makes its way to the kidneys. The kidneys then balance the elements in the blood and the substances and water (filtered blood), which the body doesn't need at that time, form the urine we pass.

Urine is just an overflow or surplus which your body doesn't need at any particular time. For example, if you drink a liter of water when you're relaxed watching a movie, you may need to take a wee once or twice. If you drink a liter of water after you completed a strenuous workout, you may not have to wee at all. This doesn't mean that the water wasn't good for you while you're inactive watching the movie, it just means that your body didn't need it at that time.

Urine is a derivative of blood and contains hundreds of components which are useful for your body. Some reasons why UT may be so effective is that it reabsorbs and reuses nutrients, hormones, enzymes, and urea. It stimulates the defense of your immune system, has a bacterial and virucidal effect and more[15]. You may have heard of soldiers using urine to apply to wounds.

You already know that your body produces antibodies. When you are ill, these antibodies are produced to counteract your illness. By ingesting your urine, you reintroduce these antibodies into your system; antibodies developed by and for your own body and illness, what more can you ask for? I've seen urine referred to as your holographic substance, so it knows exactly what your body needs.

Have you asked yourself "if it is so good, why haven't most people heard of this?" Take a moment to ask what's in it for the pharmaceutical and medical industry if more people were aware of UT? Can you see them advertising a product which won't produce a profit?

Considerations

Let's take a minute to discuss side effects. Like other detox methods, in the initial stages, there could be symptoms related to your body's releasing of toxins such as headaches, nausea, fatigue, rashes, and diarrhea, all which typically disappear in a short time.

Had I known about UT just six months before learning about it, it would have saved me pain in two specific instances. First, I was eaten alive by mosquitos at night while traveling deep in the Peruvian Amazon. I mostly slept in a hammock, and to say I was fresh meat for the mosquitos, was a severe understatement. For several weeks after returning, my bites were still with me and those that had healed left scars.

About a month later, I was traveling from Easter Island, Chile to Brasilia, Brazil. The total flight time with connections was more than 35 hours. Shortly after departing Easter Island, a finger was feeling a little sore, like when you rip a cuticle. At first, I thought nothing of it, however within a couple of hours in flight, it started to swell, and as time went by it grew larger and became very painful. Then, I noticed the same was happening to a finger on my other hand.

During one of my connections, I went into an airport pharmacy, by this time my fingers were turning green; yuck, I know. Although they provided some topical ointment, they advised it wouldn't do much and I should get to a doctor as soon as possible, and that's exactly what I did after arriving in Brasilia. I would have gladly used UT, had I known of it at the time!

If you'd like to try UT, you don't have to dive in by drinking it straight away. Pace yourself as you see fit.

- If you have a poor diet with lots of processed foods, sugar, meats, etc., you may want to make some changes here first. For example, if your urine is very dark this may mean you're not consuming enough water.

- Try taking a little bit of fresh urine and rubbing it into your skin, like your thighs and knees. If you apply it straight away, without getting it on your clothes, it will not smell.

- If you'd like to take another step, take a drop or two of fresh urine and place it under your tongue, or massage it into your gums.

- A further step would be to take a sip or two.

If you decide to take your urine orally, it's suggested to:

- Use the first urine in the morning, midstream. Midstream because your body may pass toxins first.

- Avoid if you've had too much alcohol the day before.

- Ensure it is fresh, not diluted or boiled.

Also ensure your genital area is clean, without any chemically produced soaps and so on; drink plenty of water throughout the day; and if you are pregnant, seek the advice of your doctor first.

As with all other techniques in this book, seek the advice of a qualified professional or medical doctor regarding your circumstances and advice on using UT.

REIKI

Reiki is love, love is wholeness, wholeness is balance, balance is well-being, well-being is freedom from disease.

– Dr. Mikao Usui

One of my favorite practices is Reiki, pronounced "ray-key" in the West. When I explain to family, friends, and others that I practice Reiki, I get really excited to hear that more and more of them are familiar with it.

I remember my first experience receiving a Reiki treatment nearly 10 years ago, two things really stood out. When my practitioner placed her hands at the top of my head, I could feel a heavy and tingling sensation, even though her hands were lightly touching.

When the session was complete, I noticed that I could breathe. In fact, I realized that prior to the treatment, I hadn't been breathing properly; my breath had been short and shallow. This for me was astounding and although I didn't even know I was getting a Reiki treatment, it was physical evidence that whatever was going on, something worked.

So, what is Reiki and how can it help you?

What is Reiki?

A simple explanation is that Reiki is a deeply relaxing hands-on technique, which reduces stress and promotes healing.

In more spiritual terms, Reiki is known as an omnipresent universal life energy, which is available to all. The word Reiki is a two-syllable Japanese term. *Rei*, means universal, spiritual consciousness or higher intelligence. *Ki*, you may remember is the Japanese equivalent to Qi, our nonphysical energy or vital life force. So, you may say Reiki is universal, all-knowing life force energy.

Reiki has been around for thousands of years and only recently has science begun an attempt to understand or quantify the results with research. William Lee Rand wrote an article in the 2005 winter volume of the *Reiki News Magazine* which outlines how Reiki is measured using magnetograms, and this is my takeaway.

As you know from previous sections, we are surrounded by electromagnetic fields. Each body organ has its own electromagnetic field and every electromagnetic field vibrates at its own pulse or frequency. When a person receives Reiki, any unhealthy area in the patient raises its frequency to the higher, healthier, frequency of the electromagnetic field of the Reiki practitioners' hands.

Were you ever in a room, on a bus or train, and suddenly somebody bursts out laughing so hard, that you and everyone in the surrounding area can't help but to crack up yourself? In my mind, it's similar in principle where you've raised your frequency to the person laughing out loud.

Where did Reiki originate?[16]

Mikao Usui, a Japanese Buddhist monk born in 1865, is credited for introducing Reiki in Japan in 1922. However, it is known that there were other similar, hands-on healing techniques being practiced at the time, both in Japan and Tibet. It is also believed that hands-on healing techniques have been practiced for thousands of years before Buddha and Christ.

From an early age, Usui practiced a Japanese form of Qi Gong called Kiko. Kiko is a combined practice of meditation, breathing, and slow-moving exercises to improve and maintain good health. It focuses the use of Ki (Qi) and healing through hands. The use of Kiko for healing uses one's own energy which can leave the practitioner feeling drained of energy.

Usui was in search of a way to heal without draining his own energy. In 1922, Usui decided to take a spiritual retreat for 21 days on Mt. Kurama, where he fasted, chanted, meditated and prayed. Toward the end of his retreat, he had a powerful and enlightening experience which enabled him to channel energy to others without draining or using his own.

He then practiced Reiki on himself and family members, and subsequently established a healing society and clinic for patients and taught Reiki to others. The Reiki practice from Usui is known as *Usui Reiki Ryoho Gakkai*. One of Usui's students was Dr. C. Hayashi who later trained Hawayo Takata, a Hawaiian of Japanese descent. Takata is credited for the spread of Reiki throughout the United States and rest of the world. Reiki has continued to evolve, and you will now find various types of Reiki teachings available.

Benefits

In today's stressed-out world, one of the greatest benefits of Reiki is to help patients relax. The most common feedback received by patients after receiving Reiki treatments is "I feel so relaxed," "I feel so calm," "I had the most restful sleep," and "I feel a sense of clarity and focus."

Reiki has been steadily gaining popularity in hospitals in the U.S. and globally. There has been more and more research, studies, and anecdotal evidence of Reiki's benefits over the past 40 years which shows Reiki can help with the following and more:

- Accelerated surgical recovery
- Enhanced well-being
- Greater self-awareness
- Improved sleep
- Pain management
- Relaxation

- Reduced side effects from radiation, chemotherapy, and medications

It can also help cope with a wide range of health conditions such as:

- Anxiety

- Attention deficit disorder and attention deficit hyperactivity disorder

- Autism

- Cancer

- Chronic pain

- Crohn's disease

- Depression

- End-of-life care and bereavement

- Heart disease

- Infertility

- Irritable bowel syndrome

- Parkinson's

We already know that we are an interconnected system mentally, emotionally, physically, and spiritually, and Reiki helps on all levels. It's a beautiful experience to see a patient release an emotional block during a Reiki session; sometimes they will recognize what they are finally letting go of, and sometimes not.

To demonstrate the removing or releasing of an energetic block-age, I'll share another personal experience I had with Reiki. During my Reiki Master Teacher training, we were learning an advanced technique for aura clearing. When it was my turn to experience this, I was laying on the table thinking, "Oh no, I don't really have any issues that come to mind". At the same time, I remember I had the same thought during my NLP training and found it was best to go with whatever pops up, no matter how small or insignificant it may seem. Just go with it, and let the sub-conscious mind do the work.

My mind was blank, however unexpectedly, my hands kept auto-matically and involuntarily going to my abdomen. I kept pulling them away, and they kept going back. Even though my mouth and mind said they didn't have anything to work on, my body said otherwise, so we went with this.

During the process, it was if my subconscious was unfolding. I was observing my body, which was now curling into the fetal position. I tried to stop it and lay straight on the table, but no, no, no, my body kept curling up as if it had a mind of its own, and it did. While this was happening, my body released intense pain and emotion; it was so hard and so deep, it felt like grief. When asked to describe what the shape was in this area of my body, I remember saying it felt like a ball, floating in water, and it felt like it needed protection.

Logically and analytically, what took place is difficult to explain. At the end of the day, I don't need to know exactly what occurred or why, what matters is that I released an energetic block and felt much lighter as a result.

ABET practitioners typically include a standard Reiki session as a part of their holistic approach to ABET. You may recall I received one during my first ABET experience.

You can also experience Reiki independent of ABET. The effects of a Reiki session will vary from person to person and from session to session. It's recommended that you find a Reiki practitioner that you are comfortable with. Do your research and ask questions just as you would any other professional provider.

QUALITY LIFESTYLE HABITS

The Chinese do not draw any distinction between food and medicine.

– Lin Yutang

Lifestyle habits are an important part of the ABET approach. It wasn't until a few years ago that I really paid attention to a saying I heard as a child, "you are what you eat." Thinking about the implications of this statement, I've come to appreciate the need for good eating habits. Now when I eat, I mostly ask myself if what I'm put in my mouth will help support or damage my health. Even if I decide to eat something that isn't good for me, it's okay; I am aware and making a conscious decision to do so. I enjoy every bite and appreciate that I have the option to choose.

Have you ever stopped to ask yourself:

- Why are the foods you eat different from the foods others eat in different parts of the world?

- Would you eat differently if you were raised by different parents or in a different region of the world?

- Why is it common for Americans to fill their drinks full of ice while in other parts of the world using ice in a drink is the exception?

- Why do you think eating meat is necessary and makes you strong when cows don't even eat meat?

- Why do some people eat cow meat and others horse meat?

- Why do you eat eggs or cereal for breakfast and not for other meals?

- Why do you have a drink with your meal?

All the answers boil down to learned habits. Lifestyle habits such as eating, are just that, habits. The good news is that habits are learned and can be changed, and new, better habits can be learned.

Instead of sharing a long list of dos and don'ts and all the scientific basis for each, I'll share some of the changes I've made over the past few years, some of which were learned after being introduced to ABET, such as no cold drinks. Many of these I gradually incorporated into my lifestyle as I educated myself, over time.

It's worth noting that what I'm sharing is my personal guide and it's not extensive. For example, I do enjoy cold foods like ice cream, I enjoy eating a burger and ribs every now and again, and I don't meditate fanatically. However, I make these the exceptions. So, with that, here we go, in no order of importance.

ABET, Acupuncture, and Traditional Chinese Medicine

Acupuncture had been on my radar for many years and I first tried it after my ABET training. I was amazed to see the acupuncturist treating the same acupoints we learned in ABET! When I named the acupoints where the doctor was placing needles on out loud, it was funny to hear him comment that he didn't recall the exact names of the acupoints, although he had known what the points were and what to treat.

Acupuncture and ABET are great ways to stimulate and activate energy and increase your immune system. You'll find some insurance plans now cover acupuncture and energy medicine as a benefit. I recently read that in Tennessee, one of the major insurance companies, BlueCross BlueShield of Tennessee, removed a prescription and addictive narcotic Oxycontin from its coverage and added acupuncture for pain relief among other conditions.

Aromatherapy, Essential Oils, and Hydrosols

Aromatherapy or essential oil therapy uses naturally extracted aromatic essences from plants, fruits, roots, and seeds. Hydrosols are steam-distillated aromatic waters from flowers, roots, plants, etc.

They are great for your overall well-being, to balance, harmonize, and promote physical and mental health, and can increase your immune system and energy levels.

There are a wide range of internal and external uses of essential oils in traditional medicines, such as Ayurveda and Traditional Chinese Medicine, and in everyday products such as soaps, lotions and cosmetics. You can easily find dedicated books on the use of essential oils in your local bookstore.

Essential oils vary seasonally and geographically based on native plants available. I've learned to become aware of the contents of my essential oils; the best is pure, undiluted, and contains no other additives.

Barefoot

Walking barefoot on cold or synthetic floors depletes your body's energy. It's best to walk around your home with shoes or slippers, unless of course your floors are made of real wood or bare earth.

Coconut Oil

I've known about the multitude of benefits of coconut oil for many years. I even tried to convert to using it more than 10 years ago. When I first purchased coconut oil, it was one that was supposed to be of top quality. I think what turned me off for so long, is that it had a coconut taste, which I didn't like.

It wasn't until I lived in Asia that I really incorporated coconut into my life. Even being back in the U.S., I've never had another coconut oil that had the same taste as my original purchase, so I assume it was that specific brand. I now use it in 90 percent of my cooking. I use it as moisturizer and hair conditioner, among other uses. I sometimes use it as a replacement to milk in my tea, albeit my first preference is coconut milk.

I even used coconut oil on my family's dog which helped to clear up a skin condition and he loves it, even when I add it to his food!

Coffee and Tea

There are numerous studies which explore both the benefits and the negative impacts of coffee, making it confusing to know whether drinking coffee is really good or really bad for our health. If you believe you absolutely cannot live without your coffee:

- Reduce your consumption and drink moderately.
- Don't drink it on an empty stomach.
- Replace your dairy additive with coconut milk or coconut oil.
- Drink a glass of water after each cup of coffee to rehydrate.

Being primarily a tea drinker myself, these are some of the changes I've incorporated:

- Where possible, I drink herbal teas. When I say herbal, I mean fresh where possible. One thing I observed in my travels is that other cultures use the live herbs and plants from the garden in their teas, not the manmade versions we purchase. For example, while I was at a homestay in Mexico, cinnamon tea was just that, cinnamon sticks in hot water. While in Tibet, they used fresh ginger in hot water for ginger tea. While I was studying ABET, I was able to make moxa tea by using the moxa leaves from the garden.

- I love my black tea and by black tea, I mean my English breakfast tea with milk and sugar. Now I substitute sugar with honey and sometimes raw, unprocessed sugar, and substitute milk with coconut milk or coconut oil. I limit my intake, most of the time, and I always drink water (at room temperature) afterward.

(No) Cold Drinks

You saw how important the spleen is earlier in the Traditional Chinese Medicine section. Cold drinks and foods weaken your spleen and digestion, which means your body may not be able to produce energy and blood. In other words, it takes more energy to warm the cold drinks to your body's temperature and slows down the body's metabolism.

I'll never forget, during my first visit to China many years ago, when I asked for water, it was served hot. Now I understand why.

Craniosacral Therapy (CST)

Craniosacral Therapy is a gentle, hands-on approach that releases tensions deep in the body to relieve pain and improve overall health. CST helps release electromagnetic energy imbalances in the body and untighten fascia tensions. (Fascia and electromagnetic energy were discussed in previous chapters).

The first time I experienced CST, I was amazed to feel energy moving in certain positions where the practitioner placed her hands.

Crossing Your Legs

For many years working in an office environment, I crossed my legs while sitting at my desk and in meetings. I later experienced some of the issues this could cause, specifically lower back pain and uneven hips. Even after the advice of my chiropractor and massage therapist, it took me years and discipline to break the habit; well it's a continuous work in progress. I still cross my legs on occasion out of comfort, however I do so with lots of internal conversation in my head as it goes against all I know.

Crossing your legs also blocks and decreases your energy. It's best to sit with your legs uncrossed and flat on the floor, even if this is not how we've been taught to sit, especially the ladies.

Deodorants

Most deodorants contain alcohol or synthetic fragrances, antiperspirants, or aluminum; these chemicals keep sweat in your body which becomes a problem as sweat helps to remove toxins via your skin, your body's largest organ.

Many years ago, I changed to using a deodorant stone made from mineral salts. I learned that you must always read the label as some still include aluminum. As a further alternative, you can also try coconut oil mixed with essential oils such as rose, citronella, kaffir lime, lavender, or your favorite oil.

Detox, Detox Bath and Fasting

Detox and nourish your body. Try the detox bath mentioned earlier and discover how your sleep quality improves, how refreshed you feel, how your energy increases and how your body shape changes. As I finalize writing this book, I've made my way back to the U.S. and I've already installed a hand-held sprayer. You can find them online or in your home improvement store, and they are so simple to install, I did it myself!

When I heard "fasting" in the past, I'd conjured painful images of starving myself without food and drinking only water for an entire week. These images are a bit dated and there are easier and friendlier ways to fast which work around our busy lifestyles, such as intermittent fasting. The benefits of fasting go beyond weight management and an increase of fat burning/fat loss, for instance, lower insulin and sugar levels.

There are many short- and long-term fasting options[17], some of which could include:

- Fasting for a window of time, for example eight, 12, 16, or 20 hours. This fast can be done for instance between

6 p.m. and 6 a.m. or noon to noon with meals taken outside the fasting window.

- Longer fasts could entail fasting for a 24- or 48-hour window once a week, such as on the weekend.
- Shorter fasts can easily be done daily, for example from 8 p.m. until 6 a.m.
- You may consider longer fasts once a week (e.g., 24 or 48 hours) or once a month (e.g., 36 hours).

Try an Ayurveda *Panchakarma* cleanse once a year. This cleanse I undertook in India was one of the best things I did for my body. It even cleans toxins from your body at the cellular level. I lost about eight pounds that I couldn't visibly see, and when I asked the doctor, he informed me the weight loss was primarily toxins in my body.

Electromagnetic Fields (EMF), Laptops, and Wi-Fi

We talked earlier about electromagnetic fields and know that some are good for us, and some which are not, may increase disease and impact your immune system. Research studies have begun to point links between EMF and diseases such as multiple sclerosis, rheumatoid arthritis, celiac disease, diabetes, autism, tumors, and brain cancer.

If you don't want to electri-fry your brain, these types of EMFs should be avoided when possible. For example, completely switch off your mobile phones, devices, and home Wi-Fi systems when you go to bed at night to reduce EMF exposure. Airplane mode is not considered completely switching off. I know it may seem hard, but it is possible to live with a real alarm clock and not a mobile device on your nightstand.

For similar reasons, ensure your body is protected from your electronic devices. For example, do not use your laptop or electronic devices on your lap, stomach, or legs (or any body part), and use earphones or a hands-free device with your mobile phone.

You may recall in my first ABET session, it was recommended for me to stop using my laptop on my lap. This was a difficult habit for me to change, mainly because I didn't want to. Although I began to limit the use of my laptop where it shouldn't be, I found months later I still had specific acupoints that were continuously weak. These did not become strong until I finally stopped placing my laptop on my legs.

Emotions and Thought Patterns

Emotions are energy that also impact our physical and mental state. In Traditional Chinese Medicine and other Eastern cultures, emotions are associated to your organs. If you have unhealthy emotions and thought patterns, these directly impact your organs and physical state and vice versa. Remember the relationship between the spleen and worry?

It's okay and healthy to have and express emotions, like grief, etc. It's when we hang on to and suppress these emotions that they become energetic blocks that contribute to physical symptoms and disease.

Find ways to resolve negative emotions and heal your emotional wounds, whether it's using some of the techniques noted such as Reiki or seeking help from others.

Every cell in your body responds to your emotions and thought patterns. So, remember to let go of destructive emotions that no longer serve you, like anger and resentment, and remember to ask and give forgiveness, including forgiving yourself. We are human after all, and we can learn something from every action we take or don't take, good or bad.

As I continued to focus on my personal development via different means such as my NLP training, my Reiki practice, silent mediations and more, my thought process became much more positive and now, energetic blocks are released more quickly and frequently. I've become a more open person as a result.

Exercise

Exercise should not be painful or stressful, nor does it have to include expensive gym memberships. Find exercises that you enjoy and which you can easily incorporate into your life. I have a lot of respect for runners but believe me I am not one! My exercise would include walking, yoga, and Pilates where possible. For a period of time, I incorporated cycling and walking to and from work a few days a week instead of spending that time in a gym or in traffic.

I was turned on to and made a believer of Pilates several years ago when I had serious issues with my lower back. My chiropractor recommended Pilates when, after many sessions, my back was not improving; Pilates absolutely did the trick!

Qi Gong and Tai Chi are on my list to learn and practice as they also help balance your body with deliberate movements, meditation, and breathing exercises.

Fats

There are good fats and there are bad fats. For many years we have been guided to believe that all fats are bad for our health, and pushed toward low-fat, no-fat products which can lead to problems in our bodies.

Bad fats such as margarine, hydronated vegetable oils, and non-dairy creamers, negatively impact your immune system where fats from healthy sources are vital for our bodies.

Natural fats contain nutrients called essential fatty acids which are needed for many body functions to build and repair; some of these can only be obtained by food and oils, for instance: wild game, avocados, almonds, pumpkins, pecans, pine nuts, unsalted sunflower seeds, rice bran, sesame, corn, sunflower, olive oils, and especially coconut oil.

Avoid hydrogenated vegetable and seed oils which have been artificially manipulated into saturated fats, called trans fats.

Fruits

We've all been taught that fruits are good for us. Did you know that fruits are easier to digest and metabolize when eaten on an empty stomach? Because of this, we were taught in ABET to eat fruit alone, not with meals; ripe papaya and pineapple are the exception.

Ideally, it's best to eat them ripe, directly from the tree. Can you remember how delicious the last piece of fruit you ate directly from the tree tasted? What a difference than the cardboard-tasting fruit we mostly buy in the grocery stores! After eating the sweet, ripe bananas in places in South America, Asia, and Ethiopia, I rarely buy bananas in the U.S. or Europe which have very little taste in comparison.

Where possible, eat organic, local, and seasonal fruits. Remember that imported, organic fruits are contaminated by the fumigation process required for imports.

There are many simple ways of washing pesticides off fruit such as soaking in vinegar, lemon juice, or using salt and water.

GMO (Genetically Modified Organisms)

There's lots of debate around GMO foods. It wasn't until 13 years ago when I read the book *Natural Cures 'They' Don't Want You to Know About* by Kevin Trudeau, that I really began to understand what GMO meant, and how harmful it is, to our bodies and our environment.

To me, GMO is like taking my DNA, manipulating it to create an artificial duplicate of me in a laboratory and calling this creation natural, when in fact it is not. The Non-GMO Project has a more detailed and scientific definition on their site which is a good source of GMO information[18].

GMOs cause health and environmental damage and have been banned in 300 regions globally. Did you know that most packaged foods in the U.S., contain ingredients which are sourced from genetically modified crops such as corn?

It's best to avoid foods which have been genetically modified.

Ginger

Ginger is a widely used Chinese medicinal herb which can help with inflammation, digestion, infections. It lowers cholesterol levels, reduces the side effects of monosodium glutamate (MSG), and much more.

I generally find that most of the ginger in the U.S. grocery stores is imported from China, which I prefer to avoid. It took extensive search to find a local market which sells locally grown ginger, and then it is occasionally available.

Honey

Prior to ABET training, I'd already begun to substitute sugar with the use of honey. What I didn't know, is that there is honey, and then there is honey.

Most commercial honeys are filtered and pasteurized which removes valuable nutrients and pollen and destroys yeast cells. Some tests found toxic ingredients, high-fructose corn syrup, and even antibodies in many commercial honeys.

Did you know that raw honey helps with your quality of sleep? It does for numerous reasons, including the fact it helps release melatonin, a body hormone that helps with sleep.

Honey is best when it is raw, contains pollen, and is neither pressure filtered nor pasteurized. Of course, where possible, buy local.

Meat

On one hand, the issue of eating meat has never been a big deal for me, and on the other, in the back of my mind, there is a question I felt I would need to address one day. It's never been a big issue, because I would eat meat as an exception, not every day and not every meal. On the other hand, I know there is the question of the humane aspect of the fact we farm animals only to kill them to satisfy our eating habits.

As my Ayurvedic doctor Dr. Sathyajith points out, all animals and beings want to protect themselves and no animal or being wants to be killed.

There is online documentary called *Food Choice Documentary*, that I found an excellent source of information. Among other topics, it outlines the dis-beliefs we have about eating meat, alternative sources of protein, and even the damage the meat industry including organic, grass-fed meats is having on our environment. For instance, 70 percent of U.S. land suitable for agriculture is used to grow crops for animals, not for humans, and it takes on average 2,400 gallons of water and 12 pounds of grain to produce one pound of beef[19].

I won't address whether eating meat is consciously right or wrong here, as, like all else, it's an individual choice. If you do eat meat, there are some considerations.

Meats, particularly red meats, are highly acidic and too much acidity in our bodies contributes to cancer, obesity, fatigue, heart disease, diabetes, and other health problems.

A great amount of energy in your body is used to digest foods. Meat, particularly red, takes much more effort for your body to digest. It's like using energy to carry a full backpack of unnecessary items for a two-hour uphill hike, when all you needed to carry was water and snacks. It's an unnecessary expenditure of energy that could be put to better use. You can hike much easier without the excess weight and your body can function better without having to waste energy digesting unnecessary foods.

If eating meat is a must for you, consider:

- Reducing the amount eaten, this includes portion control
- Eat grass-fed meats and avoid meats which are injected with growth hormones, steroids, and antibodies
- Consume red meat with horseradish or strong mustard to stimulate the liver and gallbladder
- Add ginger to meat to help digestion
- If you want more protein, try nuts, seeds, and spirulina

Meditation and Tibetan Breathing

Good breathing and meditation are great ways to reduce stress as they calm and relax the body and mind. Good breathing reduces blood pressure, stimulates digestion, and helps clean your body of toxins.

Yoga Nidra is an excellent relaxation and meditation technique.

Microwave

I stopped using microwaves years ago as it depletes your food of nutrition. Instead, I warm things up in a toaster oven or on the stove. It's quick and easy.

Milk & Calcium .

Have you stopped to think that humans are the only species that drink milk after weaning and that we're the only species that drink the milk of other animals? We are led to believe that milk is one of the best sources of calcium. We are told that milk is good for our bones when, in fact, it contains phosphates which reduces the absorption of calcium.

If we stay with the thought "you are what you eat and drink," we must know that we consume all the artificial growth hormones that are injected into cows. When I underwent an Ayurvedic body cleanse in India, they embraced this concept. They treated their cows as holy animals with the knowledge that we consume in the dairy products of milk, curd, etc., what the cow consumes. These cows had a significant amount of space to roam free, ate the organic Ayurvedic plants and herbs grown on-site, and were well looked after; they were even supported spiritually with prayer and blessings.

Compare this description of how their cows are treated versus how cows for commercial consumption and milk production are treated in the West; which do you think is best for your body? I can tell you, you would never recognize the taste of milk from these cows! It is nothing like the milk we drink in the West!

Our cows graze on the beach from early morning, fulfilling their natural habit. They are hand washed with water so that they feel more touched and loved by humans, creating a bond. As a result, when the cow gives milk, with the same motherly love as it does to its calf, it is more nourishing for us. Their cows graze on naturally growing grass and graze under the sun which is important for their health. In ancient scriptures, the hump on bulls and cows absorb energy from the sun.

They are not given supplements. They are given natural and organic powdered lentils, grains, millet, corn, ground-nut, cotton seed, sesame seed, small portions of jaggery, sea salt, and Himalayan salt.

They are milked only in the morning and only two nipples are milked, leaving the rest for the calf.

– Dr. Sathyajith, Ayurveda Yoga Village

Pasteurized milk destroys its natural enzymes. I recently found a local supplier of raw cow milk and it's crazy that their label must contain the words "not for human consumption" as nothing bad has happened to me by drinking it.

You can obtain calcium via other healthier sources such as: almonds, broccoli, fresh butter, collard greens, kale, moringa leaves, mulberry tea, oranges, sesame seeds, spinach, and fresh, live-culture yogurt.

Photo biomodulation-Near Infrared

PBM-NIR therapy uses near infrared wave lengths to penetrate the body to deliver energy to cells, stimulating healing and relieving pain. Infrared energy is invisible and penetrates deeper than red light therapy, enabling it to reach muscles, bones, soft tissue, and joints.

A few known applications of PBM-NIR are for pain, inflammations, and autoimmune disorders. It also increases energy, promotes cell regeneration, boosts metabolism, stimulates white blood cell production, and increases circulation.

Neck and Abdomen

There are many wind-sensitive acupoints on your body including your neck and abdomen. It's best to keep these covered, especially if you have a fan, wind, or air conditioning hitting these spots. I've spent many years in hot climates such as Florida and

Thailand, and the air conditioning in cars, restaurants, and buildings make you feel like it's winter inside, so I typically carry a scarf wherever I go. High-collared shirts are also useful.

Nuts and Seeds

Nuts and seeds are rich sources of amino acids and essential fatty acids, when eaten raw and freshly harvested. Vegetarians can easily get all essential amino and fatty acids which meat eaters get from animal protein by eating a handful of raw nuts and seeds per day.

Some of the most nutritious nuts and seeds are almonds, pecans, flax, sunflower, and pumpkin seeds. I usually have a bag of mixed nuts, seeds, and dried fruit, especially in my car. Eating just a small bit makes me feel incredibly full and find I don't want to eat much for a longer period between meals.

Poo

When was the last time you looked at your stool, really looked? Believe it or not, it can tell a lot about your health.

If you recall in the TCM section, there is an ideal time in which each organ functions best; for the large intestine that time is between 5 a.m. and 7 a.m. If you are not passing stool regularly around this time daily, you may have a problem.

Healthy stool should be firm and large like a German sausage. If your stool is regularly thin, like a pencil, this may be an indication of colon problems or hemorrhoids. If you are regularly constipated or your stool is regularly small and pebbly, it may be an indication you need to drink more water or eat more fiber.

So, you can see there is more to poo then just eliminating waste. Make a point of observing your stool and if you regularly find you are constipated, or it's irregular, seek professional advice.

Processed Foods

What's natural about processed foods? Nothing! What's good about processed foods for your body? Nothing!

It's simply best to reduce or eliminate processed foods as much as you can.

Read Labels

Be aware of what's in the food you are buying by reading labels and ignoring the marketing which grabs your immediate attention. Have you noticed there is nothing natural in the ingredients of many products labeled as such?

When I was younger, I used to say to myself that if I had money, I'd stuff my kitchen cabinets with food. Now that I pay more attention to what I'm buying, my shelves are nearly empty with minimal foods in a box.

Salt

Salt is another topic which we've been educated to believe is not good for us. Quite the opposite, it is a vital nutrient and we cannot function without it. Low-salt/no-salt diets can cause problems such as dehydration, edema, fatigue, kidney and liver problems, and more.

The main problem is that most of the salt we consume is processed and contains products such as aluminum and silicate, and is stripped of nutrients. Given the way we are polluting our oceans, some sea salt now includes plastic particles.

The best salt for consumption is good-quality sea salt, Celtic salt, and Himalayan salt.

Seafood

Fish is also an acidic food, but more easily digested than meat.

Did you know shellfish and reef fish live in polluted, shallow sea beds which filters the junk we throw into the seas? We are not only what we eat, we are also "what we eat, eats." This is one reason since ABET that I limit any intake of seafood/shellfish such as shrimp.

Wild fish is by far a better choice than farmed; however, given our rate of pollution and over-commercialization, wild fish is becoming more difficult to find.

Like most commercially raised land animals, farmed fish are raised in overcrowded and restricted containers, are given antibiotics, and are fed harmful products such as genetically modified corn. Tests have shown that farmed salmon is one of the most toxic foods in the world and even include pollutants such as a synthetic rubber chemical used in the production of tires. Yuck, is this what you want to put in your body?

Sleep

Sleep is important for your body and mind to recuperate and regenerate to stay healthy. Many of the foods we eat and many of our lifestyle habits impact our sleep, like sleeping with Wi-Fi on, reading emails in the middle of the night, and eating snacks before going to bed. If you have problems with sleep, try some of the techniques outlined in this book, such as Tibetan breathing and Reiki.

Many cultures recommend sleeping following nature's clock. For example, going to sleep and waking with the sunset and sunrise. I remember my Ayurvedic doctor saying something to the effect of humans are the only ones that wake up to an alarm clock, and you never see cows sleeping in or hitting the snooze button. I also notice my family's chickens instinctively come out of their house at the crack of dawn and go in and huddle together at sunset.

Other suggestions include:

- Go to bed before 10 p.m. or 11 p.m.; follow nature's rhythm

- Sleep with the lights off

- Put your mobile phone, television, and electronic devices away 30 minutes prior to going to sleep

- Turn off all Wi-Fi devices before going to bed

- Take a teaspoonful of honey before bed

- Drink a glass of water before bed

- Use an essential oil like lavender on your pillow

- I also use self-Reiki to help fall asleep

Slow Down and Stop Eating When Full

How often do you eat in front of the television or your tablet? How often do you eat with an electronic device, like your phone or e-reader, in your hand? How often do you eat while reading emails? How often do you eat at your desk? How often do you sit down and eat, and only eat without other distractions?

When it comes to eating, one of the greatest lessons I've learned from Buddhist and Indian cultures is to slow down and pay attention. This means eating without distractions, paying attention to what and how you are eating, and enjoying every bite. I should also add, chew thoroughly, if not, you make your body work harder and why would you want to expend energy unnecessarily? 115

A few years back I was working on a project in Brazil for two months. This office had a policy of no eating in the office which meant that everyone took a full lunch hour break, outside the office to sit and eat. During that time, I ate three full meals a day, ate larger lunches than I normally would, and actually lost weight when I wasn't trying to. I put the weight loss down to making time, slowing down, and enjoying what I was eating, especially not eating lunch while working at my desk.

Additionally, stop eating when your stomach tells you it's full. I am guilty of this often myself; I've always been told I don't eat enough, or I'm told, "you eat like a bird". The best approach is to listen to your body, it knows best what it needs.

I remember as a child I spent a summer with my step-grand-parents. As a child, I always heard, "you're too skinny" and that summer my step-grandmother offered to give me one dollar for every pound I gained by the time I left. She encouraged me to eat bread and sugar every day. Can you imagine, I was only about eight years old?!

Enjoying your meal without distraction and stopping when full can assist you with weight maintenance.

Sugar

Sugar is a dangerous substance, especially white, refined sugar, as it suppresses the immune system and the release of growth hormones in the pituitary gland, the main regulator of the immune system. Cancer cells just love sugar. Sugar:

- Is nutritionally naked.
- Causes cavities by taking away calcium from inside the teeth.
- Causes intense cravings as it leaches potassium and magnesium.
- Is addictive; Do you know how much sugar is hidden in the foods and drinks you consume?
- Is the main cause of diseases like diabetes, candidiasis, and obesity.
- Can cause behavioral problems, especially in children, such as violence and learning impediments.

When your body consumes more sugar than it can use for energy, the liver converts the extra sugar into triglycerides and stores them as fat or to produce cholesterol.

Of course, not all sugars are the same; some are good and some bad, so what can you do?

- Become aware of your sugar intake.
- Read food labels to identify hidden sugars.

- Avoid artificial sweeteners and processed foods.

- Reduce or eliminate soft drinks and artificially sweetened fruit juices.

- Eat more (ripe) fruit.

- Cook more meals at home to control what you eat.

- Use natural sweeteners such as stevia and raw honey.

- Enjoy your sweet treats like ice cream, cookies, and chocolate as the exception, not the rule.

Tongue

Have you looked at your tongue lately? What color is it? Do you have cracked lines? Do you have teeth marks on the side? Do you have spots? Is your tongue greasy? Does your tongue have a film?

I now pay attention to the condition of my tongue, it's an excellent indicator of my health. Tongue diagnosis is a specialty most TCM doctors are trained in. Remember in my ABET session I had teeth marks which was an indication of dampness. My teeth marks have gradually lessened as I've changed my eating habits.

Urine

Like your poo, pay attention to your urine as it can tell a lot about your health. It should be clear to pale yellow in color. If you have problems starting or stopping, painful urination, discolored urination (e.g., red, green, orange), leaking or dribbling, waking up too frequently at night to urinate, urinating too frequently, etc., these may be indications of a problem.

Urotherapy (UT)

You already read the benefits of UT.

Vegetables

I think we were all told as kids to eat our veggies as they would make us strong, just like Popeye. Vegetables are one of the most alkalizing foods; they contain fiber, and as we read earlier, many are good sources of calcium.

You may recall in my first ABET session, I was advised to eat cooked vegetables. This conflicted with what I had been taught, that eating raw vegetables was the best for you. In my case, given the weak spleen, slightly cooked vegetables were better because they are easier to digest.

Where possible, eat organic, local, and seasonal vegetables. Remember that imported, organic vegetables are contaminated by the fumigation process required for importation.

Water

Like honey, there is water and then there is water. You may recall during my first ABET sessions, the water I drank was tested and found that I would need to drink nine bottles. When I chose a better-quality water, my body only required two. So, not all bottled water is the same.

In Western countries, we think our tap water is safe, when in fact numerous toxins can be found, such as fluoride[20], chlorine, lead, mercury, chemicals, pesticides, herbicides, and more.

Water is in every cell and tissue in your body. It keeps things moving in your body and flushes out toxins. It regulates body temperature and lubricates joints and organs.

Our bodies are made up of more than 70 percent water. Did you know these facts?

- Your brain is made up of about 75 percent water.
- Your blood is more than 50 percent water.
- Your muscle weight is more than 70 percent water.

So, wouldn't you agree that water is crucial to your health?

If you are thirsty, your body is already dehydrated. Insufficient water leads to dehydration; it can contribute to back pain, asthmas, allergies, diabetes, weight gain, headaches, sleeplessness, arthritis, depression, and much more.

The best water is water which still contains the essential nutrients—spring and well water if you have access, mineral water or water filtered via a carbon filter. I recently learned that cilantro is a great natural water filter, for example place a handful of cilantro in two liters of water and it will absorb heavy metals and harmful chemicals[21]. Remember that using reverse osmosis water systems not only takes the bad stuff from your water, it also takes the good stuff such as the minerals and vitamins your body needs.

The amount of water each person requires depends on one's constitution, physical activities, the season, food habits, etc. Below are some general guidelines that are good habits to incorporate for a healthy lifestyle:

- Drink two glasses of water when you wake up in the morning.

- Drink one glass 30 minutes before meals (helps digestive system better absorb nutrients).

- Avoid drinking during meals or within 30 minutes after.

- Drink one glass, one hour before going to sleep.

- Drink a glass of water after every cup of tea, coffee, and glass of alcohol (to rehydrate).

- Try placing fresh fruit in your water for flavor instead sodas and fruit juices.

- Drink warm or room temperature water, never cold.

- Drink fresh coconut water, where available. I loved drinking from freshly cut coconuts in many countries I visited. Delicious!

One final note I always keep in the back of my mind is **"don't let the exceptions become the norm**." Back in the U.S., I've had to constantly remind myself of this, as it's easy to get out of the mindset of good lifestyle habits. Before you know it, too many exceptions, too often, become the norm.

All lifestyle habits are choices we make, and we can choose to make new habits. If it seems overwhelming, do what you feel is right for you and your body. After all, how many times have you read one day that something is bad for you and at the same time other studies show the same is good.

For me, it's all about balance, moderation, and sustainability. Take baby steps, if you need to. Some of my new habits were developed over a period of time. Remember my coconut oil story? For example, you may choose to stop drinking cold drinks this month, and in a month, you may cut back on your portion of meats. Start with drinking one glass of water in the morning and increase it later. Another baby step could be to vary the vegetables on your plate, as a guide, fill your plate with the colors of the rainbow.

Every day, every hour, every moment is an opportunity to make a new habit, a new choice.

As you saw from my first ABET sessions, lifestyle changes were a significant part of the ABET approach. ABET

practitioners may suggest lifestyle changes to help your body promote self-healing and help you feel better.

As they say in TCM, let your food be thy medicine.

HOW ABET HAS HELPED OTHERS

Now that you know about ABET, I'd like to share with you a few stories about how ABET has helped others. When I had the idea of this book, I approached Cory about some of her experiences and most of these stories are a direct contribution from her[22]. For privacy, I have not used full names and have removed most personal details.

Mr. J was a young, strong, and adventurous executive when at the age of 46 he suffered a stroke that left him completely paralyzed on the entire left side of his body.

During the six years after his stroke, Mr. J tried all he could with Western, traditional, and natural medicines, including spiritual activities, without any change in his condition. This led him to try ABET.

He was unable to physically smile, his left hand was a claw which he could not move, he could not walk in a straight line, he dragged his left foot, he wasn't able to drink without spilling, he would miss words while reading, and had motion sickness.

During four months of ABET, several techniques were used, lifestyle changes recommended, and specific exercises were given. These included acutouch, magnet therapy, moxibustion, Reiki,

Tibetan breathing, and more. He was also taught Reiki, so he could treat himself.

Mr. J had many ups and downs during his four months of ABET, as his body began readjusting itself and he began exercising unused muscles. He began to experience steady progress and improvement, some of which included:

- Being able to lift his left leg when sitting and walking
- Being able to smile
- Being able to gradually lift his hand and independently move it
- His motion sickness disappearing
- His headaches disappearing
- The color of his skin become less red and more natural looking
- Moving his left thumb, which also became softer and suppler
- Rotating his left arm

After two months he also had significant psychological shifts such as feelings of well-being, and he was able to begin sexual relations again.

After four months, all the challenges he faced were lessened or completely gone. He subsequently moved to another city, started working, and began to live a normal life again.

Within a year, Mr. J was completely recovered, and advised he had made more progress in the four months of ABET and Reiki than in the six years after his stroke.

* * *

Mr. E was energetic and physically active when he suffered a stroke at 47 years old. He had many healthy lifestyle habits such as playing multiple sports, rarely drank coffee or alcohol, avoided processed foods, sugar, MSG, and other unhealthy foods. He was a high-level executive who traveled frequently, worked long and hard, earned a good living, but had little time to spend it.

His stroke impacted his entire right side of body, speech, and memory, and as you'd imagine, had psychological implications, especially when two days after his stroke, his doctor advised he would not live to see the end of the week.

One month after his stroke, he was advised he would never walk and talk again, and just prior to beginning ABET, he was advised by his specialist that he had come as far as he could and would live the rest of his life with his limitations.

Two weeks after his stroke, Mr. E spent three months in the hospital where he began rehabilitation, including physiotherapy, and occupational and speech therapy. He subsequently searched for other natural therapies such as acupuncture, shiatsu, Tai Chi, yoga, reflexology, and meditation. He spent time with a psychologist and coach, and eventually turned to ABET.

Mr. E was in wheelchair for just over a year and fortunately recovered most of speech and memory just 30 days after his stroke. While he was improving when he began ABET, he still had physical and cognitive issues, including weakness on his right side, difficulties in walking, tiredness, and more.

Mr. E had 32 ABET sessions over a four-month period where various ABET techniques were used, his food habits were adjusted, and specific exercises were given. He was trained in Reiki, so he could give himself Reiki treatments. Throughout ABET:

- His sleep began improving
- He became more aware of the minute changes in his body
- He no longer experienced car sickness
- His foot came back to its natural color
- His energy levels became more stable
- He was able to reduce other therapies
- He was gradually able to move his fingers independently and stretch his arms
- He became less critical of himself and less angry at his situation
- He started feeling good and began to feel more associated with his body and body parts

One month after his ABET was completed, he moved to another country, and within six months he had a girlfriend, was walking fully and living a normal life again. As you can imagine, he was thrilled with his progress.

* * *

Ms. D is a strong and robust 35-year-old, and the way she came to ABET is quite an interesting story.

She was visiting Chiang Mai, Thailand with a friend. The day before leaving the country, Ms. D and her friend were out wandering on their motorbike and were surprised when they happened to land at Asian Healing Arts Center. The funny part or synchronicity about this story is that during her time in Chiang Mai, Ms. D had been trying to correspond with Asian Healing Arts Center, without success, and while wandering the back roads with no intention, happened to come across it.

Given Ms. D's imminent departure from Thailand, she was given her first ABET session that day and returned two months later for a subsequent six ABET sessions, Reiki, and ABET training.

Ms. D had serious problems with asthma and allergies. She constantly used an inhaler and was frequently rushed to the hospital when she couldn't breathe, where she would be given cortisone injections. She had knee pain, very dry, red, and bloodshot eyes, and she did not sleep well.

Included in Ms. D's ABET sessions were moxibustion, Reiki, cold packs for a detox bath, and these suggested lifestyle changes. She was to:

- Keep her neck area covered with a scarf and her face covered, particularly when riding her motorbike or in direct access to air conditioners and fans.
- Go to bed before 11 p.m.
- Drink wine with food, not on an empty stomach.
- Drink quality water.
- Take a spoon of honey before sleep.
- Eliminate MSG.
- Not use laptop on her lap.
- Drink specific herbal teas to help cool down her internal body.
- Turn Wi-Fi and phone off while sleeping.
- Reduce intake of red meats.
- Do Tibetan breathing twice a day.

From her very first ABET session Ms. D saw immediate effects:

- Within 30 minutes of sitting on a cold pack, her eyes went from bloodshot red to clear white. Subsequently, she rarely had red eyes after her second ABET session.
- Her knee pain disappeared.
- She was sleeping well through the night.

- She rarely used her inhaler and in the six months after her first ABET treatment, only went to the hospital once.

- She had better focus and felt full of energy.

- She felt she could breathe again.

What I also found amazing was she was no longer afraid of insects and sleeping without a light, and after her Reiki level one and level two training, she no longer had a desire to smoke.

Ms. D lost a significant amount of weight and her life was completely transformed in so many ways, including her career and spiritual paths.

* * *

Mr. G was diagnosed with Parkinson's at the age of 59 which mostly affected the right side of his body. He used various medications to help control his symptoms and began ABET seven years after his diagnosis. His symptoms included:

- Tremors and lack of control of his right arm

- A very stiff claw hand

- Being unable to walk straight; his leg was thrown when walking

- Blurry eye sight, even with prescription glasses

- Lack of energy, especially in the morning and afternoons

- Sleeping only three to four hours per night

- Consecutive sneezing for up to an hour during the night
- No sense of taste or smell
- Regular constipation
- Anxiety and depression
- Hearing his heartbeat in one ear
- His face being heavily masked with little expressive movements

Mr. G's time in in Thailand was for three weeks where he had ABET sessions five to six days a week and received Reiki training. Throughout that year, he gave himself daily Reiki treatments, continued with Tibetan breathing and still showed the following improvements:

- His hand tremors subsided.
- His eye sight had improved.
- He had increased energy, especially in the mornings.
- His sleep increased to six hours per night.
- His sneezing at night stopped.
- His sense of taste returned.
- He was no longer constipated.
- He no longer heard his heartbeat in his ear.
- He had small improvements with his facial expressions.
- His medications (self-medicated) were reduced with no increase of Parkinson's symptoms.

During his second set of ABET sessions a year later, he:

- Increased his self-Reiki treatments to two or three times per day
- Did Tibetan breathing when taking his medications
- He provided himself moxa treatments when he felt stiff

After these ABET sessions, he felt stronger, was walking better, and was able to sleep eight to nine hours per night continuously. He continued to have fewer hand tremors with reduced medication, was feeling more optimistic, and less anxious and depressed.

* * *

Mr. F, an alert 85-year-old entrepreneur, sought ABET for his diabetes in October. His blood sugar levels were 260 without medication and ranged from 150 to 180 with medications, and his blood pressure was 130/65 with medications. He had pain in his leg, used a walker, was taking 10 different types of medications, and got up to urinate every two hours at night.

Mr. F had several ABET sessions over the course of 18 months which included moxibustion, moxa footbaths, Tibetan breathing, Reiki treatments, and Reiki training. He also made the following changes to his food habits:

- Eliminated cold drinks
- Reduced or eliminated candies and sweets

- Eliminated margarine

- Eliminated MSG

- Replaced table salt with sea salt

- Introduced barley/job tears to his food options

- Ate fruit only between meals

- Incorporated coconut oil into cooking

After Mr. F's first ABET session, he stopped using his walker, began using a walking stick and over time, began walking independently without any support.

His blood sugar levels eventually dropped to the range of 130 to 150 and his leg pain disappeared. His doctor reduced his medications and his daily insulin checks. He slept better and only had to get up a couple times a night to urinate. Mr. F felt more alive and lived a higher-quality life until 88 years old.

* * *

There are times when those who seek ABET are so far along with their disease, that the only thing you can do is support and comfort them, and help ease the physical, emotional, and psychological pain. ABET and Reiki can play a key role as seen by the stories below.

* * *

Mr. S, 70 years old, came for ABET in November. He had been active and in good physical shape; he had good eating and drinking habits, such as drinking lots water and freshly squeezed juices, eating fruits, nuts and vegetables, and did not use processed sugar or eat meat.

He went to see his doctor as he had pain below his left ribs. After various tests, he was advised he had lymphoid and throat, and possibly bone marrow cancer, pending additional test results.

Mr. S was seeing a Traditional Chinese Medicine doctor who referred him for ABET. Along with the TCM herbs, medicines and acupuncture sessions provided by his TCM doctor, he began receiving standard ABET sessions, which included slight changes to his food habits, specific herbal teas, a change in the quality of water he was drinking, and Reiki treatments.

ABET and Reiki helped to reduce the pain he had, helped him sleep better, helped with his bowel movements, and even the tumor in his large intestine had reduced in a short time.

Alongside TCM and ABET, he also experimented with other treatments, such as taking DMSO, dimethyl sulfoxide, which is supposed to help with side effects of chemotherapy treatments, among other things.

Sadly, his cancer was so far along when discovered, that by the end of February he could no longer swim and play golf. In November, his TCM doctor confirmed his cancer was incurable, and by early March confirmed he was too weak to take any additional treatments.

From March until his passing in April, he continued to receive Reiki treatments, which helped him relax, sleep better, and be as comfortable as he could under his circumstances.

* * *

Mr. P was a 46-year-old who worked six days a week with only a short half-hour lunch break. When he came for ABET in February, he had been diagnosed with stage four liver cancer, was in a wheelchair, and was very weak after having undergone a series of chemotherapy treatments.

Mr. P had a total of 17 ABET sessions over an eight-month period. In the first months, he began to steadily improve. For instance, by his second ABET session, he began walking without a wheelchair. Throughout his ABET sessions, he stopped eating meat, drank specific herbal teas, made changes to his eating habits, was given herbs by a TCM doctor, took time off work, and received regular Reiki treatments.

He steadily improved, his pain reduced significantly when walking, his burping stopped (previously a big problem), he was able to sleep well, and began having regular bowel movements.

Unfortunately, during the last month or so, Mr. P went back to his previous habits, such as eating meat and working six days a week. By August, his condition began to deteriorate and by September he passed away.

* * *

A more recent and personal experience is with a dear friend, Mr. M, 80 years young. Shortly before my arrival back to the U.S., he had undergone surgery for prostate cancer. His physical and mental state had suddenly declined after his surgery and the outlook was not positive. This was a major adjustment, which caused him significant stress. I was able to support him with Reiki treatments, and although I was sad to see his condition, I was very grateful to be with him in the last few weeks of his life. It was beautiful to see how he embraced and looked forward to his Reiki sessions and to see the comfort it brought him during such a difficult time.

CONCLUSION

The art of medicine consists in amusing the patient while nature cures the disease.

– Voltaire

The natural techniques and lifestyle habits shared are just a taste of the many that are available to us all. These have served me well at different points along my journey, physically, mentally, emotionally and spiritually. Some of the direct benefits of ABET for me include:

- I'm more aware of how to conserve and use my (Qi) energy.

- I'm aware of how the relationship of Qi, the spleen, dampness and the environment impacted the fatigue I used to feel.

- I'm more conscious of how certain lifestyle habits directly impact my health, like cold drinks.

- I haven't had a cold in over two years and if I remotely feel one starting to come, the feeling quickly passes, and the cold does not materialize.

- I have not used an over-the-counter drug in over three years. For minor aches such as headaches and cramps, I now use magnets or other ABET tools without the use of drugs.

- The persistent cough I used to experience, has become less frequent.

- I no longer buy expensive moisturizers, lotions, or hair conditioner, instead I simply use coconut oil. If I want a scent, I'll add an essential oil like lavender.

- ABET has provided me more natural options in my personal healthcare toolkit and more tangible tools that I can leverage to help others on their journey.

Some of my key learnings along this journey include:

- **We are a whole being.** It's important to take care of our mental, physical, emotional, and spiritual well-being. Neglecting one aspect is like having a broken leg of a table, resulting in an imbalance.

- **Everything is interconnected.** We are connected to and dependent on the world around us. The environment is just one aspect. For instance, if we pollute the water, there will no longer be fish or water to sustain us. If we pollute our air, we will have trouble breathing. If we inject hormones into animals, spray crops with harmful chemicals, or consume genetically modified foods, there is a direct and harmful impact to our health. If we allow the bee population to be destroyed, we will destroy a main pollinator of the plants that produce our foods. If we care for our environment, plants, animals, and so on, they will care for us.

- **Nature provides.** Urine therapy is an excellent example of nature's intelligence. The most effective therapies available come from nature. What are drugs after all? Many drugs are based on ingredients from plants and nature which have been manipulated and synthetically reproduced.

- **Treating a symptom does not cure the problem**; finding and addressing the root cause will. If you live on the fourth floor of a building and have a clogged pipe, trying to unclog the drain on the fourth floor may not resolve the issue if the cause is on any of the floors below you. It's the same with your health.

- **Listen to your body.** We may feel bombarded with instantaneous access to information at our fingertips, however if we take the time to listen to our body, we can make the best choices for us as individual beings. Your body will tell you when to stop eating. It will tell you which foods it wants.

- **Cookie-cutter solutions don't work for all of us.** We are unique beings in mind, body, and soul. So, do what's right for you because what may work for me, your family or friends, may not work for you, and what works for us today, may be different tomorrow.

- **We perceive the easiest changes to be the hardest.** You may recall that one of changes I perceived to be difficult was to stop using my laptop on my lap (e.g., while lying in bed or sitting on the sofa). It was an easy change to make, I just didn't want to give up the convenience.

- **We are responsible for our own choices**, so take ownership. You are the only person responsible for your decisions, choices, and their respective outcomes.

- **There is room for Western, natural, and complementary therapies.** The challenge we have begun to face is that our right to choose is being taken away by government regulations. Physicians are being trained and forced to push chemical-based therapies on us. Become aware, educated, and act to ensure you have a right to choose the therapies you want for you and your children.

Just like our cars will run more smoothly and last longer if we regularly service and maintain them, our body will take care of us, if we take care of it.

There is a saying that "your body is your temple," however many of us treat it like it's a garbage bin. Most of us would feel much better just by making small lifestyle changes. Why not make positive lifestyle changes now while you are able to do it freely and easily instead of waiting until you're too ill or it's too late to have a positive impact? Would you wait until your car is completely dead to change the oil or have it serviced?

I hope you've found these ABET techniques useful and that you choose to incorporate those that resonate with you into your life and share them with the world to make it a better place for all.

Thank you and namaste.

REFERENCE

My Journey and Why This Book

1. *Causes* by Madeleine Innocent, Two legs and Four Whole Health, twolegsandfour.com.au/

Dr. Thanh Van Le

2. Information regarding Dr. Le was provided by Cory Croymans from Asian Healing Arts Center (AHAC), during and after ABET training.

Cory Croymans and How ABET Saved Her Life

3. New Life Foundation, under the patronage of H.R.H. The Princess Mother. Based in Chiang Mai, Thailand, this charity organization helps underprivileged Thais with mental or physical disabilities. asianhealingartscenter.com/new-life-foundation.htm

What Is the O-Ring test?

4. Quotation from bdort.org/

5. These two sites are useful for information regarding Dr. Y. Omura and BDORT. http://drgadol.com/bi-digital-o-ring-test-bdort/ and bdort.org/

Techniques to Restore Balance and Promote Healing

6. ABET training handout: The Piezo Trigger Technique, Asian Healing Arts Center

7. Moxa: The information below was provided to us in ABET. I was unable to find the original source of the studies, so I have placed them here as a reference only.

*   Studies show that the white blood cell count begins to increase immediately after moxibustion and reaches a peak eight hours later and is then maintained for 24 hours. This number remains elevated for four or five days after treatment. The white blood cell count almost doubles with moxibustion, but when applied continuously for six weeks, the increase is sustained for up to three months after moxibustion is discontinued.

*   Studies found that subjects who had an average hemoglobin ratio of 78 percent just before direct moxibustion, the ratio increased steadily to reach a peak of 90 percent in eight weeks.

*   When applying moxibustion continuously for 15 weeks, it takes 22 weeks for the red blood cell count to return to what it used to be before moxibustion.

*   It also shows a substantial increase in the following blood components: the sedimentation rate of red blood cells, platelet count, the speed of blood coagulation, blood

calcium, blood glucose count, the capacity to produce antibodies

- Because of stronger effects on the overall biochemical changes, especially in blood components and immune system, moxibustion is more effective for chronic diseases of internal organs.

Detox Bath

8. The term "detox bath" was originally termed by R. Khalil and L. Baker, authors of The New Detox Bath, which can be found on their website pureinsideout.com.

9. Details of Mr. Louis Kuhn's story can be found in Neo-Naturopathy, The New Science of Healing, by Louis Kuhne, 1917.

10. France Guillain's story was outlined in a handout provided in ABET training by Asian Healing Arts Center. It is referenced from a translation called The Deviating Douche (DD) by France Guillain. The translator advises the document was a translation of a 180-minute recording of a seminar which was given by France Guillain in 2003. The translator's name was not provided in the AHAC document. You can view or request this document on liveyouryellowbrickroad.com or via Asian Healing Arts Center, Chiang Mai, Thailand.

11. Guillain explains her view of the fascia system in more detail in the recording referenced above.

12. The New Detox Bath, by R. Khalil and L. Baker and their website: pureinsideout.com.

13. Variations of the detox bath can be found in the handout mentioned in reference 10 above and in a handout provided in ABET training from Asian Healing Arts Center, called "DD Benefits of Cold Pack. The New Detox Bath, by R. Khalil and L. Baker is also a great resource and can be found on their website: pureinsideout.com/.

Divine Nectar

14. You can read more about Christy's story in her book *Your Own Perfect Medicine.*

15. Reasons why UT may be so effective were covered in depth in ABET training. Additionally, *The Golden Fountain* by Coen van der Kroon, is a great resource to learn more. It has an entire section of possible reasons, including those I listed and more with detailed and thorough explanations.

Reiki

16. There are slight variations and beliefs about the origins of Reiki, and I believe the most common and widely taught comes from William Lee Rand, Walter Lübeck, and Frank Arjava Petter, who extensively researched Reiki. *The Spirit*

of Reiki, The Complete Handbook of the Reiki System, is one of their published resources.

17. I found this blog article on fasting to be an easy and informational read on fasting: dietdoctor.com/intermittent-fasting

18. The Non-GMO Project defines GMO as "...living organisms whose genetic material has been artificially manipulated in a laboratory through genetic engineering. This creates combinations of plant, animal, bacteria, and virus genes that do not occur in nature or through traditional cross-breeding methods."

"Most GMOs have been engineered to withstand the direct application of herbicide and/or to produce an insecticide. However, new technologies are now being used to artificially develop other traits in plants, such as a resistance to browning in apples, and to create new organisms using synthetic biology. Despite biotech industry promises, there is no evidence that any of the GMOs currently on the market offer increased yield, drought tolerance, enhanced nutrition, or any other consumer benefit." nongmoproject. org/gmo-facts/

19. Food Choices Documentary , (youtube.com/watch?v=6h-JNayG6dxk), foodchoicesmovie.com/ . Note that these links were available when I accessed outside the U.S., and subsequently not available when I accessed in the U.S.

20. Many of us were taught as children that fluoride was good for your teeth. I used to look forward to those fluoride tablets that made your teeth red! Instead, studies show fluoride has been linked to thyroid problems, ADHD, damage to the pineal gland, and more. Some countries now ban fluoride in water. Here are a couple of articles on fluoride and water: globalhealingcenter.com/natural-health/5-good-reasons-you-should-avoid-fluoridated-water/ and globalhealingcenter.com/natural-health/12-toxins-in-your-drinking-water/.

21. https://wisemindhealthybody.com/anya-v/cheapest-way-clean-up-tap-water/

How ABET Has Helped Others

22. All stories, excluding Mr. M, were provided by Cory Croymans, Asian Healing Arts Center.

RESOURCES AND SUGGESTED READINGS

A Short Introduction to Traditional Chinese Medicine Concepts

There have been many articles and books written on Traditional Chinese Medicine. One of my favorites is *Between Heaven and Earth: A Guide to Chinese Medicine* by Efrem Korngold and Harriet Beinfield.

More on Qi: http://acuhealing.com/tcmtheory/whatisqi.htm

Techniques to Restore Balance and Promote Healing

A good read on magnet therapy is: *Magnet Therapy*, second edition, by William Philpott, Dwight Kalita, and Linwood Lothrop.

Detox Bath

More on fat cells and heat: A 2013 article in *Science Now* magazine titled "Fat Cells Feel the Cold, Burn Calories for Heat," by Elizabeth Norton, states: "Transforming fat cells into calorie-burning machines may sound like the ultimate form of weight control, but the idea is not as far-fetched as it sounds. Unexpectedly, some fat cells directly sense dropping temperatures and release their energy as heat, according to a new study." sciencemag.org/news/2013/07/fat-cells-feel-cold-burn-calories-heat

If you read French, two of France Guillain's books on the detox bath are:

Les Bains Dérivatifs, 1995

Le Bain Dérivatif Cent Ans Après Louis Kuhne, 2000

France Guillain's website: bainsderivatifs.fr/en/

Divine Nectar

There is a great analogy in the book *The Golden Fountain* by Coen van der Kroon. The author refers to a dam and explains if the water rises over a certain level, the surplus flows away through the floodgates. It doesn't mean the surplus water is useless.

For more information on UT, you may find the following reads useful:

Your Own Perfect Medicine by Martha M. Christy

The Golden Fountain by Coen van der Kroon

The Water of Life by John W. Armstrong

Urine Therapy: Natures Elixir for Good Health by Flora Peschek-Bohmer and Gisela Schreiber

Modern Medical and Scientific Aspects of Auto Urine Therapy by Oztin: curezone.org/forums/am.asp?i=1437074

Quality Life Style Habits

Your Body's Many Cries for Water by F. Batmanghelidj, MD, is a good read if you'd like to learn more on how important water is for your body.

The Truth About Cancer documentary is excellent, https://go.thetruthaboutcancer.com/

YOUR OPINION MATTERS

Your Opinion Matters

Thank you for reading *Natural Healing Techniques, Get Well and Stay Well with Asian Bio-Energetic Therapy.*

If you've enjoyed this book, please help support us authors by placing a review on Amazon, Goodreads, Barnes & Noble, or your favorite site.

Reviews will help others find this book so they can enjoy and learn as you have done. They will also let us know how we can do better on the next book.

Thank you!

SOCIAL MEDIA

Stay in touch and share your experiences.

Learn more about ABET, Reiki, and other natural techniques and general well-being.

Join us on:

 LiveYourYellowBrickRoad.com

 @LiveYourYBR

 @LiveYourYBR

 @LiveYourYBR

Also visit Asian Healing Arts Center:

 asianhealingartscenter.com

 @soonreikichiangmai

ABOUT THE AUTHOR

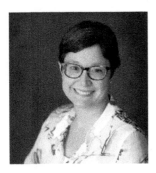

Joanne Klepal is a certified Asian Bio-Energetic Therapy practitioner, Reiki Master Teacher, Master Practitioner of Neuro-Linguistic Programming (NLP) and Coach and Master Practitioner of Timeline Therapy™. She has practiced, coached, and trained ABET, Reiki, and NLP in England, India, Thailand, and the U.S.

A global wanderer, traveling to more than 50 countries, she has resided in England, Southeast Asia and the U.S., and has recently made her home in the Florida panhandle.

For more information about Joanne, please visit: liveyouryellowbrickroad.com.

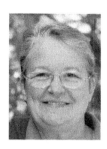

Cory Croymans was born in Belgium and has spent the past 43 years in Southeast Asia. She has trained in Asian Bio-Energetic Therapy, Aromatherapy, Homeopathy, Reiki, Traditional Chinese Medicine, Craniosacral Therapy and Thanatology. She is the founder of Asian Healing Arts Center in Chiang Mai, Thailand where she practices and teaches Asian Bio-Energetic Therapy, Reiki, and Aromatherapy.

For more information about Cory or to locate an ABET practitioner near you, please visit: asianhealingartscenter.com.

A portion of net proceeds will be donated to charities of author(s) choice such as the New Life Foundation[3].